DESIGNER BABIES:

WHERE SHOULD WE DRAW THE LINE?

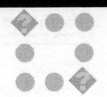

DESIGNER BABIES:

WHERE SHOULD WE DRAW THE LINE?

Institute of Ideas
Expanding the Boundaries of Public Debate

Ellie Lee
Veronica English
Ann Sommerville
Agnes Fletcher
Juliet Tizzard
Professor John Harris
Josephine Quintavalle

Hodder & Stoughton

A MEMBER OF THE HODDER HEADLINE GROUP

DEBATING MATTERS

Orders: please contact Bookpoint Ltd, 130 Milton Park, Abingdon, Oxon OX14 4SB. Telephone: (44) 01235 827720. Fax: (44) 01235 400454. Lines are open from 9.00 - 6.00, Monday to Saturday, with a 24 hour message answering service. Email address: orders@bookpoint.co.uk

British Library Cataloguing in Publication Data
A catalogue record for this title is available from the British Library

ISBN 0 340 84835 9

First Published 2002
Impression number   10 9 8 7 6 5 4 3 2 1
Year   2007 2006 2005 2004 2003 2002

Typeset by Transet Limited, Coventry, England.
Printed in Great Britain for Hodder & Stoughton Educational, a division of Hodder Headline Plc, 338 Euston Road, London NW1 3BH by Cox & Wyman, Reading, Berks.

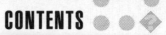

CONTENTS

PREFACE
Claire Fox

NOTES ON CONTRIBUTORS

INTRODUCTION
Ellie Lee

Essay One   **DRAWING THE LINE: THE NEED FOR BALANCE**
Veronica English and Ann Sommerville

Essay Two   **MAKING IT BETTER? DISABILITY AND GENETIC CHOICE**
Agnes Fletcher

Essay Three   **'DESIGNER BABIES': THE CASE FOR CHOICE**
Juliet Tizzard

Essay Four   **LIBERATION IN REPRODUCTION**
John Harris

Essay Five   **BETTER BY ACCIDENT THAN DESIGN**
Josephine Quintavalle

AFTERWORD
Ellie Lee

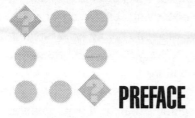

PREFACE

Since the summer of 2000, the Institute of Ideas (IoI) has organized a wide range of live debates, conferences and salons on issues of the day. The success of these events indicates a thirst for intelligent debate that goes beyond the headline or the sound-bite. The IoI was delighted to be approached by Hodder & Stoughton, with a proposal for a set of books modelled on this kind of debate. The *Debating Matters* series is the result and reflects the Institute's commitment to opening up discussions on issues which are often talked about in the public realm, but rarely interrogated outside academia, government committee or specialist milieu. Each book comprises a set of essays, which address one of four themes: law, science, society and the arts and media.

Our aim is to avoid approaching questions in too black and white a way. Instead, in each book, essayists will give voice to the various sides of the debate on contentious contemporary issues, in a readable style. Sometimes approaches will overlap, but from different perspectives and some contributors may not take a 'for or against' stance, but simply present the evidence dispassionately.

Debating Matters dwells on key issues that have emerged as concerns over the last few years, but which represent more than short-lived fads. For example, anxieties about the problem of 'designer babies', discussed in this book, have risen over the past decade. But further scientific developments in reproductive technology, accompanied by a widespread cultural distrust of the implications of these developments, means the debate about 'designer babies' is set to continue. Similarly, preoccupations with the weather may hit the news at times of flooding or extreme weather conditions, but the underlying concern about global warming and the idea that man's intervention into nature is causing the world harm, addressed in another book in the *Debating Matters* series, is an enduring theme in contemporary culture.

At the heart of the series is the recognition that in today's culture, debate is too frequently sidelined. So-called political correctness has ruled out too many issues as inappropriate for debate. The oft noted 'dumbing down' of culture and education has taken its toll on intelligent and challenging public discussion. In the House of Commons, and in politics more generally, exchanges of views are downgraded in favour of consensus and arguments over matters of principle are a rarity. In our universities, current relativist orthodoxy celebrates all views as equal as though there are no arguments to win. Whatever the cause, many in academia bemoan the loss of the vibrant contestation and robust refutation of ideas in seminars, lecture halls and research papers. Trends in the media have led to more 'reality TV', than TV debates about real issues and newspapers favour the personal column rather than the extended polemical essay. All these trends and more have had a chilling effect on debate.

But for society in general, and for individuals within it, the need for a robust intellectual approach to major issues of our day is essential. The *Debating Matters* series is one contribution to encouraging contest about ideas, so vital if we are to understand the world and play a part in shaping its future. You may not agree with all the essays in the *Debating Matters* series and you may not find all your questions answered or all your intellectual curiosity sated, but we hope you will find the essays stimulating, thought provoking and a spur to carrying on the debate long after you have closed the book.

Claire Fox, Director, Institute of Ideas

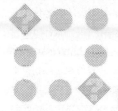

NOTES ON THE CONTRIBUTORS

Veronica English is the Deputy Head of Medical Ethics at the British Medical Association. Her role is to provide ethical advice for doctors in response to enquiries and to prepare guidance and reports on a range of ethical issues. Before joining the BMA in 1994, she worked for seven years in the regulation of infertility treatment with both voluntary and statutory regulatory authorities.

Agnes Fletcher is a disabled woman with an inheritable impairment, who has been thinking, talking and writing about genetics and disability for more than ten years. In 1999, she conducted a survey of disabled people's attitudes to developments in genetics (Genes Are Us?, RADAR, London). She works for the Disability Rights Commision.

John Harris is the Sir David Alliance Professor of Bioethics at the University of Manchester, a member of the United Kingdom Human Genetics Commission and of the Ethics Committee of the British Medical Association. His essay, published here, is the result of research spanning a number of years and related ideas have been published or will be published as the following: *Clones, Genes and Immortality* (Oxford University Press, 1988), 'Rights and Reproductive Choice' in John Harris and Søren Holm (eds) *The Future of Human Reproduction* (Oxford University Press, 1998), 'The Concept of the Person and the Value of Life' in *Kennedy Institute of Ethics Journal* 9, 4, 1999, 'Is there a Coherent Social Conception of Disability' in the *Journal of Medical Ethics* 26, 2, April 2000, 'Cloning and Balanced Ethics' in

Iain Torrance (ed.) *Bioethics in the New Millennium* (St Andrews Press, 2000), and 'Reproductive Choice' in *Encyclopaedia of the Human Genome* (Nature Publishing Group, 2002).

Ellie Lee teaches sociology and social policy at the University of Southampton. Her research interests lie in the areas of the sociology of social problems and policy developments in the areas of the regulation of reproductive technology, and mental health. She is commissioning editor for the law section of the *Debating Matters* series.

Josephine Quintavalle co-founded Comment on Reproductive Ethics (CORE) in 1994, a public interest group working to encourage balanced debate on issues associated with human reproduction, and has hosted or assisted in many bioethics conferences, consultations and briefings both nationally and internationally. She is an English graduate and is on the board of the Centre for Bioethics and Public Policy (CBPP).

Ann Sommerville is Head of the Medical Ethics Department at the British Medical Association where she has worked since 1987. She is particularly interested in the interface between medicine, ethics, law and human rights.

Juliet Tizzard is director of Progress Educational Trust, a charity set up to promote the benefits of reproductive and genetic science. She is also editor-in-chief of *BioNews*, a web-based news and comment service.

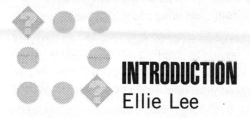

INTRODUCTION
Ellie Lee

The term 'designer baby' has become part of everyday language. But what is a 'designer baby'? Adam Nash was labelled the world's first example of this kind of child. The embryo that became Adam was genetically selected, using preimplantation genetic diagnosis (PGD), to ensure it was free from the gene fault for the serious and sometimes fatal condition of Fanconi's anaemia, suffered by Adam's sister Molly (the details of this technique are described later). After Adam was born without the condition in August 2000, he became donor to his sister, providing her with blood that more than doubled her survival chances.

What made this child a 'designer' child was that, according to many commentators, he represented a precedent, where the possibility of parents using science to choose aspects of their offspring's genetic make-up, had become a reality. This, according to such opinion, was a dangerous development. It could lead to a situation, perceived as negative, where parents could 'design' children with a variety of genetic traits.

In February 2002, the possibility that a 'designer baby' would for the first time be created in the UK was announced, when the Human Fertilisation and Embryology Authority (HFEA) authorized the use of PGD by a couple from Leeds. The regulation of the use of PGD by the HFEA is discussed in more detail later, but the Authority's ruling in this case was widely considered a 'landmark' decision.

The couple concerned, Shahana and Raj Hashmi, were given the go ahead to use the technique to select an embryo free from the gene fault for the blood disorder thalassemia, and which would have genes that could allow a baby born as a result to become a bone-marrow donor to his or her brother. The Hashmi's existing child suffers from thalassemia, and the request to use PGD was made by this couple, since a suitable bone-marrow donor that could save their existing child's life could not be found. In the immediate wake of this ruling, it was reported that six more couples announced their intention to apply to use PGD for similar ends. As with the Nash case, in the Hashmi case too, the term 'designer baby' appeared in commentaries where the potential difficulties and 'ethical problems' allegedly thrown up by this application of PGD were debated.

As Veronica English and Ann Sommerville argue in the opening essay of this collection, the term 'designer baby' is therefore not a neutral description of a child born following the use of a reproductive technology – for example, PGD. Rather, it is a deliberately pejorative term which conveys the idea that the use of such technology is, or has the potential to be, dangerous or problematic. And discussion of 'designer babies' is almost always accompanied by the argument that there is a need for restrictions on the further development and use of reproductive technology. The notion of the 'designer baby' carries with it the demand for 'lines to be drawn' – for laws to be made or policies tightened – to prevent or at least restrict practices which can enable prospective parents to 'design' their children.

The purpose of this collection of essays is to debate the merit of such concerns about PGD and related technologies. Are there good reasons to be worried? And do lines need to be drawn? Both those who ascribe to this point of view and those who do not have contributed to this book. Our hope is that through their essays, they make a clear and convincing case for or against the use of reproductive technology and for or against further regulation of its use and future development. On the basis of their arguments, readers can decide for themselves where and whether they think lines should be drawn. The aim of the remainder of this introduction is to provide some background to the essays that follow, by summarizing the *modus operandi* of the technologies discussed in the following pages and the legal framework that currently regulates their use.

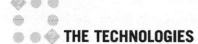

THE TECHNOLOGIES

PREIMPLANTATION GENETIC DIAGNOSIS (PGD)

This technique is discussed by all contributors to this book and has been at the centre of the debate about 'designer babies'. It came into use in the late 1980s and, for the first time, created the possibility that embryos could be selected or discarded before a pregnancy is established on the basis of whether a gene fault is present. It brings together two technologies: *in vitro* fertilization (IVF) and genetic testing. In IVF, fertilization takes place outside a woman's body, as sperm and egg are put together in a laboratory, to form an embryo. This technology was developed in the first place to treat infertility. Couples unable to conceive through sexual intercourse alone could be assisted to do so through IVF. In PGD, the use of this technique is different. Instead of transferring embryos directly to the prospective mother's womb, in the hope that a pregnancy will result, in PGD embryos are first tested for faulty genes.

A couple using PGD will undergo some interventions similar to those used in normal IVF. The woman will be given hormone injections, to stimulate the ovaries. This means that, unlike in a normal menstrual cycle where only one egg ripens and is released at ovulation, a number of eggs mature, which can each be artificially fertilized. When the eggs reach the right size, as with IVF, they are collected using ultrasound guidance. A semen sample is obtained from the woman's partner at the same time (in regular IVF, if the cause of infertility was diagnosed as related to the quality of the sperm, donor sperm would be used at this stage). The eggs are placed in an incubator and the sperm added to the eggs, to begin the process of fertilization. This happens at around four to six hours after egg collection and the fertilized eggs are grown in the laboratory for two or three days. At the end of this time, the embryo will have developed to comprise eight cells and is about one-tenth of a millimetre in size. In regular IVF, it is at this stage that up to three embryos are transferred to the womb. In PGD, genetic testing happens first and only those embryos without certain genes are transferred.

At present PGD is used mainly in relation to certain diseases where the cause of the illness is a change in a single gene. In these instances, a single cell of the embryo can be tested, and presence or absence of the gene fault that causes the disease detected. Disorders of this kind that have been tested for so far include cystic fibrosis, sickle cell anaemia, Huntington's disease, beta thalassemia and familial adenomatous polyposis coli (a form of bowel cancer). PGD has been used by those with a family history of these disorders, to avoid the birth of further children with these conditions. This list of conditions will extend in the future, as research identifies the specific gene fault involved in more single gene disorders.

Some genetically linked diseases can be tested for where they are sex linked – that is carried only by females. With these conditions, a female can be a healthy carrier of the disease, because of the presence of two X chromosomes. Males, however, because they have just one X chromosome (and one Y) will be affected by a fault on the X chromosome and will therefore experience symptoms of the disease when they are born. With such disorders, an embryo can be tested, and only female embryos transferred. In theory any X-linked disorder could be tested for in this way. At present, X-linked disorders which are commonly tested for are duchenne muscular dystrophy, haemophilia A, severe combined immunodeficiency and Fragile X syndrome.

The causes of many common diseases, such as heart disease, diabetes and Alzheimer's disease, are currently unknown however. These diseases are caused by a complex relationship involving a number of genes and environmental factors, not well understood at present. At the current time, therefore, the range of diseases that PGD can be used for is limited to a small number. Although it may be possible to do so in the future, characteristics such as height or weight cannot be tested for because such traits are, as with many common diseases, very complex. The question of whether and how they are influenced by genes is as yet unanswered. The issue of genetic enhancement, discussed in this book, thus concerns possible future developments, rather than existing practice.

Where PGD can be used, embryos where no faulty gene is evident are transferred to the womb, in the hope that a pregnancy will be established. A maximum of three is used. The other embryos with faulty genes can then be used for licensed research or are left to perish, which usually takes place in the course of a few hours.

PRE-NATAL TESTING

Another technique discussed in this book is pre-natal testing, which in fact comprises a number of different tests, carried out on women who are already pregnant. Tests vary, in that some provide an estimation of the *chance* that a fetus has a particular condition, not whether it actually has. Other tests are diagnostic – they indicate whether a particular fetus *actually has* a specific condition. Some tests have been around for many years, while others are newer, and some tests are now routine – pregnant women will usually undergo them unless they request not to – while others are used for 'high-risk' groups only. The issue of decisions for or against abortion, where pre-natal testing indicates the presence of disability of some kind in the fetus, forms a contentious area of discussion in this book.

Ultrasound

Throughout pregnancy, women will have ultrasound scans, some of which are diagnostic while others are not. Early in pregnancy (at around 12 weeks' gestation) women will routinely have a scan, the purpose of which is to confirm a live pregnancy, accurately determine the age of the fetus and see whether the pregnancy is single or multiple. At this stage, however, ultrasound cannot determine whether there are defects or abnormalities present, unless they are extremely serious. A further ultrasound at between 18 and 20 weeks is conducted, to check the fetal anatomy for developmental problems. In the course of this examination certain defects, for example of the spinal cord and head and heart, may be identified.

Nuchal translucency scan

This test is offered at 10 to 14 weeks, but is not available at all NHS hospitals so, if required, may have to be done privately. It involves conducting a detailed ultrasound scan (a high resolution scan) to detect markers that may be indicative of Down's Syndrome. These include thickening of the layer of fluid behind the fetal neck. Research suggests that this test is fairly accurate at predicting the risk of Down's Syndrome.

Maternal blood tests

Tests based on maternal blood are routinely offered to pregnant women at 15 to 18 weeks' gestation. These work by measuring the amounts of substances produced by the fetus in the mother's blood sample. In combination with the woman's age, weight, and length of pregnancy, the measurement of the level of these substances is used to estimate the chance of the fetus having certain conditions (such as 1 in 300, that is, of 300 babies born, one will have a particular condition). A raised level of a chemical called AFP indicates that the fetus may have a spinal cord defect such as spina bifida. The 'triple test' is a blood test for Down's Syndrome. It measures for low levels of AFP and also higher than normal levels of a hormone called hCG and of the hormone oestriol, all likely to be present where a woman is carrying a fetus with Down's Syndrome. These tests are not exact however. A raised risk indicated through blood tests does not diagnose the presence of a disability in the fetus. If the risk is assessed as high, the woman may be offered further tests, for example, amniocentesis.

Amniocentesis

This test is routinely offered to pregnant women over 35 and may also be offered to those assessed as high risk, through blood tests. It is used to diagnose Down's Syndrome (it is almost 100 per cent accurate) and also other conditions such as Tay-Sachs. The procedure involves taking fluid from the sac surrounding the fetus, by inserting a needle, guided by ultrasound, through the abdominal wall. Cells from the fetus present in this fluid are then tested. This test cannot be carried out before 15 or 16 weeks' gestation and carries a risk of about 1 in 100 of triggering miscarriage.

Chorionic villus sampling (CVS)

CVS also tests fetal cells and can be carried out between nine and 11 weeks' gestation, but carries a slightly higher risk than amniocentesis of triggering miscarriage. It involves analysis of a small piece of tissue from the placenta, which contains fetal cells, because the fetus and placenta develop from the same initial cells. The cells are gathered through a small tube passed through the cervix or by inserting a needle through the abdominal wall. Unreliable diagnoses are occasionally obtained and amniocentesis may be offered to clarify the result.

Cordocentesis

This samples fetal blood cells, obtained by inserting a needle guided by ultrasound into the umbilical cord. This test is similar to CVS, but because fetal blood cells are collected, results can be obtained more quickly. It is carried out from 18 weeks' gestation.

THE LAW

PGD AND THE LAW

There is no law that specifically regulates the use of PGD. Rather, it is regulated through the Human Fertilisation and Embryology Act 1990 (HFE Act). This Act regulates all activities related to human embryos outside the body – their creation, use through the provision of IVF services or for research and their storage through freezing. Under the HFE Act, research on human embryos is prohibited after 14 days.

With regard to the provision of IVF services (including PGD) clinics have to obtain a licence from the Human Fertilisation and Embryology Authority (HFEA), the body that oversees the implementation of the HFE Act, if they are to offer such services. Centres which offer IVF are subject to annual inspection by the HFEA. The only specific restriction concerning access to PGD, placed on licensed centres by the HFE Act, is that an assessment must be made by the centre of those wishing to access the service. According to section 13(5) of this Act: 'A woman shall not be provided with treatment services unless account has been taken of the welfare of any child who may be born as a result... and of any other child who may be affected by the birth.' The interpretation of what constitutes 'the best interest of the child' is, however, left to medical discretion. Whether the request of a particular couple or individual for PGD (or IVF) is accepted is determined by the view of the clinician concerned.

This section has been interpreted by some as an encouragement to clinicians to 'screen out' 'undesirable' potential parents.

In addition to a licence to provide IVF, centres carrying out PGD must also hold another licence issued by the HFEA, which deems them able to provide the genetic testing involved in the procedure. This licence is only issued when the HFEA is satisfied that the staff are proficient at carrying out the procedure.

The issue of which genetic disorders and conditions (or, potentially, attributes) centres can screen for is decided by a licensing committee of the HFEA. It decides on a case-by-case basis. To date, no genetic disorders that can be tested for have been ruled out. However, following a process of consultation in 1993, a ruling was issued that testing for sex selection on non-medical grounds is not permissible. This ruling was reconfirmed in 2000, when the HFEA was asked to reconsider its ban on non-medical sex selection by a couple named Alan and Louise Masterson, whose three-year-old daughter had died in a bonfire accident. Parents to four sons, this couple sought to use PGD to sex select, but their request was refused. In justifying the continued ban, Ruth Deech, chair of the HFEA, stated that: 'The public do not like, and we do not like, the idea of designer babies.'

PRE-NATAL TESTING AND THE LAW

There is no law that regulates the provision of pre-natal testing of pregnant women. The law that can be considered relevant, however, is the Abortion Act 1967 (as amended) since, following the diagnosis of a genetic or other condition in a fetus, a woman may consider, or request, termination of pregnancy.

Under this Act, up to 24 weeks' gestation, it is legal for a pregnancy to be terminated as long as two doctors agree that its continuation constitutes a threat to the physical or mental health of the woman concerned or that of her existing children. Where the fetus is diagnosed as at 'substantial risk of serious abnormality', however, this time limit does not apply. Since some tests to diagnose conditions in the fetus are carried out late in pregnancy, it has been deemed legally acceptable for the time limit that applies for abortion in all other circumstances (other than where the life of the woman is at risk) to be waived. In 1999, 89 abortions were carried out on this ground after 24 weeks' gestation. In total, at all gestational stages, 1,813 pregnancies were aborted where abnormality was diagnosed in the fetus, including, 329 abortions for Down's Syndrome and 434 for disorders of the nervous system.

While pre-natal screening is not subject to legal regulation, its practice is informed by guidelines issued by relevant professional bodies. The Royal College of Obstetricians and Gynaecologists, for example, has good practice procedures for pre-natal screening and diagnosis, which guide its members. These state that good practice means those involved in these procedures must ensure that women and their partners are 'aware of the benefits and risks involved with each test', that the tests are 'only undertaken with the knowledge and consent of the woman' and that women and their partners 'feel free to exercise whatever options they choose'. The question of whether adequate information is provided, and whether freedom of choice exists in practice where pre-natal screening and diagnosis are offered, are significant areas of debate for contributors to this book.

It is against this technological and regulatory background that those who have contributed to this collection make their case. For Veronica English and Ann Sommerville, the main issue is the need for balance in the debate. They argue that, on the one hand, it is important not to overstate the novelty of attempts by parents to influence their children's health or characteristics before birth or traduce and misrepresent their motivation for doing so. On the other, they contend there are well-founded concerns regarding reproductive technologies, in particular those which focus on the quality of the relationship between parents and 'designer' children, and those which construe reproductive technology as a form of discrimination against disabled people.

This theme of whether PGD, and pre-natal screening in particular, are anti-disability technologies and should be restricted for this reason is pursued by Agnes Fletcher and Juliet Tizzard. For the former, the lives of disabled people are undermined by these technologies and on this basis their use by prospective parents should be restricted. For the latter, such concerns are misplaced, and it is possible for society to both respect the rights of disabled people and allow prospective parents to choose whether or not to have a genetically impaired child. The main concern for Tizzard, which she contends is sidelined in most current debate, is lack of access to PGD and its high cost, which may prevent potential parents who need it from accessing treatment.

Like Juliet Tizzard, John Harris believes there to be few dangers posed by reproductive technologies. He contends that, in a society that values freedom, unless there are ethically compelling reasons for denying access to these interventions, people must be able to choose for themselves. A simple dislike, or even revulsion, at the choices made by others is not enough to justify restricting choice. For Harris, even in the case of non-medical sex selection and the future possibility of genetic enhancement for intelligence or talents, such compelling reasons do not exist. An argument against this case for freedom in procreation, made through a defence of the positive value for parents and society as a whole of accepting natural outcomes in pregnancy, is made by Josephine Quintavalle, in the final essay.

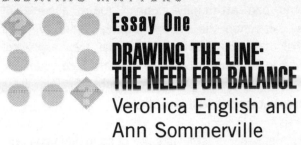

Essay One

DRAWING THE LINE: THE NEED FOR BALANCE

Veronica English and Ann Sommerville

The views expressed herein are those of the authors and not those of the British Medical Association.

> Step forward to a dinner party in 2025. Somebody mentions the amount that the Smiths have paid to make sure their next daughter has blue eyes. Wouldn't it have been better spent on making her musical?
>
> (Editorial, *The Economist*, 14 April 2001)

Throughout history, people have searched for ways of enhancing their offspring, according to their perceptions of desirability. Some hope for physical attractiveness or, like the hypothetical Smiths, for children with blue eyes, while others want particular talents, such as musical ability. Only two methods have existed for achieving this: by careful selection of a reproductive partner or by improving the environment in which the children would develop, with good nutrition and training in specific skills. Neither method offered certainty of outcome but could only shorten the odds a little. However careful the calculations of prospective parents, their ability to tip the balance strongly in favour of a talented, attractive child remained low. This was emphasized by the playwright George Bernard Shaw, when an admirer suggested that a child possessing a combination of his wit and the beauty and grace of the dancer, Isadora Duncan, would be an asset to society. Shaw allegedly replied 'but have you thought, madam, of the ghastly possibility that the child might have her brains and my face?'

Nowadays, parents can artificially control many aspects of reproduction. They can control the size and timing of their families. Where there is a risk of a serious sex-linked disorder, they may select the child's gender to avoid the disability. In industrialized countries, people tend to have few children but invest much effort in raising them, focusing on quality rather than quantity.

'Quality', however defined, is still largely dependent upon the vagaries of natural reproduction. While techniques have evolved to remove some of the perceived impediments to perfection (by interventions from pre-implantation diagnosis to plastic surgery and the panoply of the cosmetics industry) parents have no guarantees of beauty or talent. They can try to encourage appreciation of music and language while infants are still in the womb but nothing can ensure acquisition of such skills. Science may offer new possibilities, but questions arise about whether limits should be set on the options open to parents.

NATURAL VERSUS SCIENTIFIC METHODS

At least since the time of Aristotle (who advised fathers to tie off their left testicle to ensure a male child) attempts have been made to enforce parental choice. Prospective parents already engage in a range of activities to influence and improve the type of children they have. Newspaper 'lonely hearts' columns indicate a high degree of pre-selectivity about the type of people individuals are willing to meet and enter into relationships with. Even if specific attributes for future children are not consciously sought, choice of partner is often influenced, at least in part, by the selected individual's perceived suitability as co-parent.

Wertz and Fletcher have pointed out that procedures such as episiotomy, use of forceps and elective Caesarean sections were introduced into childbirth at the beginning of the last century 'from a desire for more perfect children and a distrust of natural processes, a view shared by both women and doctors at the time' (*Clinical Obstetrics and Gynaecology* 36(3), 1993, p.543). Women take folic acid prior to conception to diminish the risk of neural tube defects. Expectant mothers seek guidance about what to eat or avoid. They eschew alcohol and medication. A burgeoning publishing empire of parenting books and magazines is subsidized by people determined to ensure the best start for their children. Such almost obsessional concern with the well-being of the developing child is tacitly encouraged.

Parental attempts at social engineering and betterment of the family do not stop there. Babies are registered early for private education to ensure a place at the school parents prefer. Children are encouraged or coerced to excel in socially respected activities: football, music and dance. How many fathers try to relive their own dreams of becoming a professional footballer through their children, with or without the child's acquiescence? Parents invest considerable time, effort and cash in attempts to produce more intelligent and socially adept offspring and the idea that we should completely abandon that aim is unthinkable.

Given that parents' attempts to select and influence certain aspects of their children's health, appearance and character is such a deep-seated human urge, and that trying to improve the outcome for our children is generally seen as a laudable aim, are there any grounds for society to discriminate between different methods for doing so? Are the haphazard and frequently ineffective 'natural' methods of modifying offspring uncontroversial simply because they are as ineffective, haphazard and as totally human as unplanned reproduction, whereas using more scientific methods suggests cold bloodedness, inflexibility or unwillingness to accept human imperfection?

THERAPY VERSUS ENHANCEMENT

Few voices in society totally object to parents using medical knowledge to avoid disabilities or, indeed, to using 'natural' measures, such as exercise and tuition, to enhance their children's attractiveness or their cognitive or athletic abilities. There appears to have long been some consensus that, although parenthood is (and probably should be) a sort of lottery, pre-emptive measures to avoid suffering and impairment in children are generally acceptable in a way that similar measures aimed at enhancement over and above 'normal' functioning are not.

This dichotomy between therapy and enhancement has been criticized by some, such as Resnik, who argues that in seeking to draw such a line, society is relying on at least 'two questionable assumptions: (1) that we have a clear and uncontroversial account of health and disease and (2) that the goal of treating diseases is morally legitimate, while other goals are not' (*Cambridge Quarterly of Healthcare Ethics*, 9, 2000, p.366). Nevertheless, a key concern about permitting new types of selection or modification which have no clear therapeutic purpose is the potential for this to increase discrimination against those who are 'different' and to create unrealizable (or undesirable) expectations for perfect children. These concerns mean we may have reason to be cautious about developments in this area of medicine.

Such caution may well be required if we consider the existing trend whereby medicine is increasingly used (in cosmetic surgery, dietary regimes and so on) simply to 'improve' the bodies of people who are not sick. It would merely be a continuation of current thinking to try to extend the use of medicine into pre-programming favoured characteristics into future children. Conformity with certain norms is valued. Parents and doctors might consider feature-altering plastic surgery for children with Down's Syndrome. Such surgery would do nothing to reduce the patient's disability apart from the disability of being perceived as different.

While homogeneity is pursued by those who are 'different', those who are the same seek to distinguish themselves from the herd. Donated gametes from certain types of donor are in great demand. Beauty queens' eggs are sold to the highest bidder as well as Nobel Prize winners' sperm (presumably, Shaw would have reminded purchasers that their children might inherit the puny body of an intellectual and the intellect of a showgirl). Routinely, women undergoing IVF with donor gametes are encouraged to state preferences regarding donor height, build, eye and hair colour. Their choices mainly match the physical characteristics of their partners – an interesting twist in the 'designer baby' debate with new technologies being used to mirror natural reproduction as closely as possible.

As a society, we particularly prize any kind of exceptional talent or beauty, precisely because such attributes are relatively rare and often require dedication and high maintenance. Many people have reservations about democratizing those attributes to the extent that they could be available to all (or at least to all with sufficient financial resources). As a recent editorial in *The Economist* stated, a common argument is that a line should be drawn 'between (welcome) medical treatment and (inadvisable) parental perfectionism' because a 'queasy feeling takes over once parents start eradicating character traits such as homosexuality, or actively selecting good genes – athleticism, tallness or high IQ.'

One valid problem some commentators have with the notion of genetic enhancement is that it deprives the individual child from deciding some matters for him or herself by imposing the previous generation's priorities. There are sound arguments for avoiding decisions now which compromise the range of choices open to people later and which they may want to take themselves. Despite the frailties and complexities of individuals' value systems, parents want the best for their offspring. Sometimes they recognize that the best might include allowing them the widest choices rather than demanding measures that restrict their children's future options. 'A child who is required to take up piano lessons by his parents can later give them up; he cannot change the fact that they made him ten inches taller' (Editorial, *The Economist*, 14 April 2001).

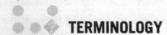

TERMINOLOGY

Terminology is central to any debate. Intentionally or not, the terms used can influence or even dictate policies. A quick perusal of any modern mass medium indicates a societal anxiety about the potential uses of genetic technology but this is often linked to the way the arguments are presented.

'DESIGNER BABIES'

The phrase 'designer babies' epitomizes the disquiet felt about attempts to control or manipulate reproduction in ways that seem to some to be unreasonable or beyond the realms of acceptability. It generally refers to genetic enhancement not therapy (although such a dichotomy is overly simplistic) and to the selection of 'trivial' characteristics at parents' whim. If a hierarchy of triviality were established, the Smith's predilection for blue eyes would probably be classed as trivial whereas their choice of a female might not, particularly if they already had male children. If they were likely to pass on a sex-linked disease, their choice of a female child would lift the decision out of the 'trivial' and into the 'suitably responsible' category.

The phrase 'designer babies' implicitly compares the child to a fashion accessory or just one more aspect of medical technology becoming a lifestyle choice, like 'designer drugs' for mood enhancement or body-enhancing surgery. The term suggests the potential to purchase a package of human attributes as easily as any other foray into 'retail therapy'. Although choice makes people feel good, this phrase is almost invariably used pejoratively. It is not applied to all attempts to manipulate reproduction. The use of preimplantation genetic diagnosis for the avoidance of disability, for example, is usually spared this label, presumably because it falls within the sphere of activity most people consider to be 'serious' and acceptable.

'ROUTINE PROCEDURE'

Pre-natal testing for disability has become such an accepted aspect of ante-natal care that it is now seen as an integral part of the planning and preparation for the birth of a child. As a result, ultrasound scans and tests for conditions such as Down's Syndrome are offered as 'routine procedures' with the expectation that women will accept them. The use of language such as 'control', 'choice' and 'reassurance' makes pre-natal diagnosis appear attractive, persuasive and the 'right' thing to do. The use of such terminology is very likely to have an impact on the perception created. Using such language to make some aspects of new reproductive technology seem 'routine' or the 'norm' makes people who oppose such interference feel that they have to work twice as hard to justify their stance.

Women often report both implicit and explicit pressure to undergo pre-natal testing. Many accept what is offered without questioning the implications. There are a number of risks arising from such routinization of pre-natal testing. One is that women who accept testing as the 'right' and 'responsible' thing to do (and do so for 'reassurance' rather than having considered the possibility of an unfavourable result) can find it particularly difficult to cope with bad news. Having been given information about a serious disability, parents must decide what, if anything to do with that information; doing nothing is no longer a neutral act.

'NORMALITY' AND 'ABNORMALITY'

While there may appear to be some societal consensus about the desirability of reducing the risks of transmission of serious disease and disability, there is less agreement about how these concepts are defined. Even the perceived boundaries of normality and abnormality, health and disease, can be seen as culture specific. Philosophers such as Foucault claim these boundaries vacillate to accommodate changing medical and societal convenience and others show how western medicine, far from embodying a coherent system, is characterized by varying cultural norms and nationally preferred diagnosis. Different diagnostic labels on different groups at different times imply that disability is a social product. Homosexuality is an example of a trait now accepted as an aspect of individual personality but which has only recently ceased to be classified as a psychiatric disorder. Individual perceptions of disability also vary. Many deaf people, for example, do not consider their condition to be a disability and some have gone so far as to say that they would support genetic testing so that they can be sure their child will also be deaf (Middleton, *American Journal of Human Genetics* 63(4), 1998, p.1175–80).

Geneticist Angus Clarke reports pregnancies where the fetus has Turner's Syndrome (resulting in infertility, shortness and sometimes in an unusual appearance) being 'terminated by couples who may be older than average and who desperately want a child but who have been told that the fetus is abnormal' (*The Lancet* 338, 1991, p.999). They lack time to gamble and may be unaware that the condition rarely causes insuperable medical problems but, in a society which apparently values a restricted range of 'normality', they find difficulty with the idea of continuing a so-called 'abnormal pregnancy'. In a study of decisions following pre-natal diagnosis, Pryde and colleagues noted a 30 per cent decision to terminate in cases of ultrasound-diagnosed abnormalities. No parents chose termination for an abnormality classified as 'mild' and only 12 per cent did so when the abnormality was defined as 'uncertain' (*Clinical Obstetrics and Gynaecology* 36(3), 1993, p.496–509). Life hangs by a label rather than a thread in such cases.

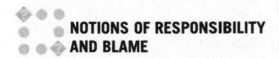

NOTIONS OF RESPONSIBILITY AND BLAME

A risk arising from perceiving pre-natal testing as the norm is that people might feel guilty or to blame for the birth of a child with a disability. Just as we often (illogically) praise parents for having talented or attractive children, might we not increasingly come to see them as failing when their offspring are less than perfect? One study indicated that obstetricians, the public and some geneticists were more prone to blame those mothers of a Down's Syndrome child who had declined screening than mothers who were not offered it (Marteau and Drake, *Social Science and Medicine* 40(8), 1995, p.1127–32). This apparent expectation that people should avail themselves of testing and then avoid the birth of disabled children could impact on the services available and influence pejoratively society's perception of disabled people. Reducing the potential for suffering through pre-natal screening has been portrayed as a personal and societal drive to eliminate certain types of individuals. We do not believe that, even if most pregnant women choose according to prevailing cultural views, a 'eugenic' society would develop. Nevertheless, for some people, abortion for disability can be more problematic, judgemental and discriminatory than the termination of a healthy fetus for more apparently trivial reasons. If a woman does not wish to be pregnant, her autonomous choice could outweigh the perceived weaker claims of the fetus. Abortion of a planned pregnancy following an unfavourable pre-natal diagnosis, however, implies a clear preference for a fetus better and more perfect than this one.

An important area of anxiety focuses on the risks, for society at large, of 'geneticization'. All sorts of legal and social concerns about personal responsibility, reward and punishment arise from the proposition that people's personality and behaviour might be determined by their genetic make-up. Increasing prominence given to genetic explanations for disability and handicap as opposed to possible social and environmental factors can also mean that less emphasis and resources are devoted to non-genetic methods of improving the quality of children's health. Focusing on genetic explanations makes it less likely that steps will be taken to augment the welfare and benefit provisions to pregnant women and children living below the poverty line, for example.

MAINTAINING A BALANCE

While there are many valid concerns about the effects of reproductive technologies, as discussed already, it is important not to trivialize the motivations of parents. Understandably, parents want to give their children a good start but they do not necessarily want perfect offspring or would reject imperfect children. Philosophical debate sometimes assumes that all decisions by intending parents are coolly calculated on the basis of data about fetal health or abnormality in line with some predefined notion of perfection. But no parent is perfect and most simply want healthy children who reflect the best characteristics of the parents themselves. Children are a form of personal continuity into the future and so must be closely linked to those aspects of ourselves we would like to see preserved into future generations. Carefully modified human templates cannot do this, no matter how perfect.

Various studies reflect the stress and anguish experienced by women accepting pre-natal diagnosis and potential termination of pregnancy. Some report bonding behaviour by parents with the unborn fetus followed by intense grief and distress occasioned by terminations. Such distress is part of the valuing of the imperfect life and a sense of bereavement about its loss. If there are misperceptions on this issue about the full psychosocial consequences of prenatal diagnosis and the alleged desire for perfect offspring, some of the ethical arguments about choice may, in fact, be superficial and unreflective of real life.

It is sometimes automatically assumed that, as soon as identification is made of a gene connected to a particular trait or characteristic, people will clamour to use genetic modification and influence that particular facet of their child's make-up. In fact, 'given the inherent limitations of the gene transfer approach to enhancement, discussion of extending such procedures to humans is scientifically unjustified' and 'where more complex traits such as intelligence are concerned, we have no idea what to do, and in fact we may never be able to use gene transfer for enhancement of such phenotypes' (Gordon, *Science* 283, 1999, p.2023). Furthermore, despite much media hype, there is no real evidence of the predicted clamour for selection of children's hair or eye colour. Perhaps the most notable exception is the very real desire for gender selection for cultural, religious or social reasons. But while some people would certainly use technology to balance their family or ensure a male first born, it is unclear to what lengths they would go to achieve that aim. As yet, it is not evident that significant numbers, in the absence of a genetically transmitted condition, would seek medical assistance and arrange conception in a clinical setting to maximize choice. This is particularly true where the selection would be carried out at the post-fertilization stage requiring the expense, inconvenience and limited success of IVF treatment.

The debate about where the limits should be set must be a balanced one. While avoiding complacency, it must also avoid automatically accepting the media's often rather sensationalist view of the likely trivialization of medicine to fulfil 'wants' rather than 'needs'. It is essential to adopt a realistic approach about what is likely to be possible and also to consider the supporting evidence (if any) for the common assumption that people wish to 'design' their children and are prepared to go to extreme lengths to achieve that aim.

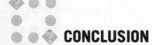

CONCLUSION

There is nothing new about dreams of perfecting an individual in whom are combined desirable physical, mental and social traits. Such fantasies are reflected in many cultures' myths and stories. For most people that is probably where they will remain – as an interesting fantasy. Nevertheless, the opportunities to try and realize some aspects of those dreams are expanding. Once technologies exist there is always a risk of a technological imperative to use them. The fear is that some people, even if not a majority, will seek to transmit some fashionable traits to their children for whimsical reasons. Parents who take extreme steps to enhance their children's skills are also likely to have rather unrealistic expectations. If they attempt to exert such control over aspects of their children's appearance and predisposition, concerns arise about the other pressures that will be applied. The implications for children who fail (by choice or design) remain to be explored. It also raises fears that the offspring will not be valued for themselves but rather as commodities or objects to serve parental needs. In the absence of suffering or disability, such a level of interference in another's life appears unacceptable meddling. As McGee points out, the popular media deal in idealized images of perfection. The perfect baby of *Cosmopolitan* or *Men's Health*, he speculates, might 'grow to be six feet tall, 185 pounds, and disease free. His IQ is 150, with special aptitudes in biomedical science. He has blond hair, blue eyes. He is aggressive [a great sportsman] but also enjoys poetry and fine wine' (*Hastings Center Report* 27(2), 1997, p.16–22). Surely such paragons would have little in common with the flawed parents who 'designed' them and might choose to only relate to other similar superbeings?

Half a century ago, the debate was rather different although the dreams of a future generation of super-fit and highly intelligent beings were the same. At that stage, however, it was envisaged that governments, rather than individual parents would be in control of the medical technology. We now look back with distaste to the debates of 1945 which urged the need for another version of 'designer babies'. Then it was seriously argued that childbearing by parents in whom 'the desired qualities are seriously lacking' should be strongly discouraged. Reproduction should be confined to those with sound health, intelligence, social usefulness, freedom from 'genetic taint' and philo-progenitiveness (desire to have many children). Women whose relatives suffered hereditary illness were to be discouraged from childbearing as were strong intelligent men who were idlers or parasites. Some may argue that the level of interference suggested by this picture of society is very different from the kind of interference parents might seek to make, but can we be certain that present or future society would handle the choices any more wisely?

Society must have reservations about facilitating the selection of 'trivial' characteristics not least because it seriously undermines the concept of unconditional love to which all children have rights. For this and for practical reasons the Smiths are unlikely, in the foreseeable future, to be able to put in an order and receive the blue-eyed female they want to select. The currently huge gulf between parents' expectations and the practically deliverable outcome is central to much concern. Nevertheless, it is too simplistic to claim that selection for medical purposes is acceptable while selection for enhancement is not. Selection and genetic manipulation to avoid serious disorders is widely seen as reasonable where parents feel comfortable about it, but it is not unproblematic. It has also long been recognized that the path from therapy to enhancement is a continuum rather than constituting a clear and obvious dividing line. In either case, care needs to be taken to ensure that pressure is not exerted on individuals to conform automatically to others' expectations (those of society or parents). Careful regulation will be needed to maintain appropriate limits. Perhaps most importantly, a preoccupation with genetics must not lead to neglect of social, political and other non-genetic solutions to the health management of future generations. For the vast majority of the world's populations, these areas are where the really important solutions have to be found.

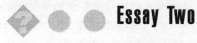

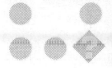

Essay Two

MAKING IT BETTER? DISABILITY AND GENETIC CHOICE

Agnes Fletcher

'Soon it will be a sin for parents to have a child that carries the heavy burden of genetic disease. We are entering a world where we have to consider the quality of our children.' So said Bob Edwards, embryologist and IVF pioneer in the *Sunday Times* on 4 July 1999.

This calls to mind medieval ideas of disability being punishment for 'the sins of the fathers'. It anticipates a culture of blame for parents of children with 'undesirable' characteristics that are preventable through preimplantation genetic diagnosis, pre-natal genetic testing followed by termination of pregnancy and somatic and germline gene therapy. How long before personal parental guilt becomes social resentment? Why should 'we' pay for 'your choice' to have a disabled child?

The international effort to map and sequence the human genome is variously driven by scientific curiosity, altruism and greed. The search for effective treatments for devastating, painful and fatal diseases is laudable – and rarely as lucrative as the patenting of gene fragments or developments of genetic tests. The search to establish and to alter the genes responsible for differences between individuals and for the extent to which an individual differs from the average is more politically and ethically charged.

Big money is involved, often spent wisely and properly. However, genetic research and technology present enormous opportunities for financial gain from exploiting the anxiety and guilt of millions, particularly in the developed world where pressure for 'consumer' choice in reproduction is increasing. Arguably, it can create more anxiety and unhappiness, by telling us something about our own or our children's future but not always giving us the opportunity to do anything about it. In the case of our 'children', it may allow us to make decisions about their future before they even have a present. This means a fundamental alteration in the relationship between parent and child.

Because of the profound consequences heralded by the possibilities of genetic engineering, it is essential to engage in an *a priori* detailed consideration, as a society, of which direction research should follow and how that research should be applied. Otherwise, these decisions are likely to be driven as much by commercial pressures and by misconceptions of factors affecting 'quality of life' as by considerations of the health and well-being of individuals or populations. Where they are driven by the natural desire of parents to confer upon their children good health and a happy life, it is important to examine the consequences of attempts to affect what is, ultimately, beyond our absolute control.

Because of the widespread use of pre-natal screening, where women who want to have children make often agonizingly difficult decisions not to have a particular child, based on predictions about its future health or characteristics, disabled people have useful experience to bring to our deliberations. This essay seeks to throw some light on the perspective this experience provides.

DISABILITY AS A SOCIAL CONSTRUCT

I am writing from a 'disability equality perspective'; that every life is of value and that the variety of characteristics among humans, our diversity as a species, has innate value. Underpinning this is an acknowledgement that everyone experiences limitations – physical, intellectual, sensory – at some point in their lives; that illness and impairment in this sense are 'normal'; and that each of us is in some way dependent on others. Indeed, for the overwhelming majority of people affected by impairments, society's response, in terms of attitudes or barriers to participation, is the determining factor affecting what is termed 'quality of life'. According to this disability equality perspective, while good healthcare is essential and should be available on the basis of need, searching for medical solutions to social ills – of prejudice, of discrimination, of failure to acknowledge and accommodate the differences among us – is wrong. At its most crude, seeking to stretch the short child to prevent it being bullied in the playground, while an understandable response by its parents, is akin to trying to whiten the skin of a black child facing similar harassment. Indeed, offering the hope of universal perfection in health terms and access for our children to the idealized average – a little taller, a little brighter, a little whiter – turns our attention from the work needed to change society to embrace the differences that exist between us all.

Disabled people point to evidence of pressure on women to take tests and to terminate pregnancies, citing for example a 1997 survey of new mothers, 'The stress of tests in Pregnancy' carried out by the National Childbirth Trust. The NCT's Policy Research Officer, Rosemary Dodds, wrote in that report: 'The technology for antenatal screening is outstripping the counselling available. Some of the parents we heard from had received crass treatment.' Indeed, some disabled people regard these pressures on women to make the 'right' choice, often portrayed as a matter of moral imperative to 'spare the suffering' of the not-to-be born, putative disabled child, as akin to selective termination on grounds of sex, race or sexuality.

Disabled people and disability organizations have demonstrated interest in the ethical and social issues raised by pre-natal genetic testing. They have discussed the issues among themselves and have sought to promote public debate. Many disabled people have a particular interest in developments in genetics, as they fear that the context in which technologies are developed and 'choice' is extended is profoundly affected by fears, myths and stereotypes about disability. Many see it as their role to warn of the divisive, marginalizing effects of developments, particularly where they move from what might widely be accepted as impairment to genetic 'enhancement'.

THE DISABILITY RIGHTS CRITIQUE OF PRE-NATAL SELECTION

Disability rights advocates have advanced the view that there is a qualitative and important difference between the decision to have a child and the decision to have, or not to have, a particular child based on a single characteristic. They believe that while these are momentous decisions of considerable personal significance, they are also decisions affected by the social context in which they are made and that they have a wider impact than the individual. To use the familiar phrase, the personal is political. Also, to reject or to attempt to choose to have a child based on a particular characteristic affects the nature of the parent–child relationship in a profound way.

Canadian academic and disability rights advocate Adrienne Asch has advanced this line of argument with particular clarity, notably in a recent collection of essays, *Prenatal Testing and Disability Rights*. Asch articulates an emotional response felt by many disabled people to attempts to screen out, via pre-natal genetic diagnosis or selective termination following pre-natal genetic testing: 'As with discrimination more generally, with prenatal diagnosis, a single trait stands in for the

19

DESIGNER BABIES: Making it better? Disability and genetic choice

whole, the trait obliterates the whole. With both discrimination and prenatal diagnosis, nobody finds out about the rest. The tests send the message that there's no need to find out about the rest.' Asch adds: 'A decision to abort based on the fact that the child is going to have specific individual characteristics such as mental retardation, or in the case of cystic fibrosis a build-up of mucus in the lungs, says that those characteristics take precedence over living itself, that they are so important and so negative, that they overpower any positive qualities there might be in being alive.'

◆◆●
●　●　 **CHANGING THE PARENT–CHILD**
●●◆ **RELATIONSHIP**

Another disabled academic, this time a British one, Dr Tom Shakespeare, has advanced the notion of the 'tentative pregnancy'; the pregnancy that is wanted but provisional until certain 'facts' about it can be established. Two things are clear – that such 'tentative pregnancies' are already widespread ('Is the baby OK?'), and that their occurrence is likely to steadily increase in many parts of the world, as increasingly sophisticated diagnostic tools become available. Indeed, while 200 years ago pregnancy was a time of enormous anxiety because of the strong risk of neither mother nor child surviving childbirth, today it seems equally fraught.

Many commentators have described how new reproductive technologies encourage a consumerist attitude towards children. At a time when society is moving towards a greater acknowledgement of the fact that barriers of attitude or environment limit the lives of many disabled people far more than any impairment or difference from the norm, a new holy grail is perceived to exist: the possibility of rooting out every 'rogue' or 'faulty' gene. If you can pay for your child's education, why not? The question, as with selective education, is whether individual parental 'choice', always limited to those who can afford it, should be fettered in any way by considerations of equality of opportunity, social cohesion or collective interests and whether such selection is positive for the child selected out or in.

Genetic intervention, particularly genetic 'enhancement', is likely to alter profoundly the relationship between parent and child. In making a wanted pregnancy 'tentative' before the 'facts' are established (absence of Down's Syndrome, musical ability), the sense is developed of baby as a product, with the 'duds' returnable under money-back guarantee.

Looking at the 'any child/this particular child' argument, Adrienne Asch believes that the decision to become a parent, if not based on the acceptance of parenting *any* child, fundamentally changes something about the parent's relationship with a particular child. If you expect to be able to determine certain outcomes, you may be deeply disappointed to find that life is still full of vicissitude and grief; that these are, quite literally, among the facts of life.

In most cases of preimplantation or pre-natal genetic diagnosis, a woman or couple wish to be pregnant at this particular time. Ending the process by discarding embryos or terminating a pregnancy happens only because of something they have learned about this particular embryo or fetus and the child it might become. Women or couples who undergo pre-natal genetic testing may consider ending a longed for pregnancy, based on a conviction that the child that would result would have a serious, negative impact on them and their families.

Some argue in response to the disability rights critique that preventing the birth of a disabled child with spina bifida is no different from taking folic acid to try to ensure the health of the developing fetus. The net result is to prevent the birth of someone with this condition. To reject this view does not necessarily imply ambivalence on the question of women's rights to abort or that having an impairment is a desirable aspect of identity, sometimes the confused interpretation of the term 'disability pride'.

For most disabled people, there is understanding of the desire for 'a healthy baby' and a very real understanding of the personal, rather than social, difficulties that can result from the experience of impairment. However, that does not imply a willingness to make the judgement that lives affected by pain, discomfort or limitation are not worth living. Each life has its troubles, its pains, its limitations, many far worse than the experience of impairment.

Again, the belief that life as a disabled child or adult is so distressing that it should be avoided if at all possible, is different from acknowledging the need for good healthcare and doing what is possible to ensure the health of the viable fetus. The decision to end the relationship begun with a prospective, wanted child and to begin again, hoping for a different child, is clearly likely to be an agonizingly difficult one. It is, therefore, important that as a society we accept responsibility for ensuring that there is a breadth of information available to parents making decisions on the basis of life with a condition that they may know little or nothing about; that there is a positive welcome and continuing support for disabled children and their families; most difficult of all, that society changes to accommodate the variety of human characteristics and experience. This latter, in particular – wider doors, low-floor buses and all the rest – is likely to benefit rather than harm most not-yet-disabled people anyway.

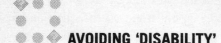

AVOIDING 'DISABILITY'

Choices regulating reproduction in the United Kingdom are mostly implemented by individual women and men, rather than as the consequence of state intervention, as in China. However, it is possible to identify considerable and increasing pressures on prospective parents that undermine the exercise of free choice.

The Nuffield Council on Bioethics, in its 1993 report *Genetic Screening: Ethical Issues*, predicted that the 'potential of eugenic misuse of genetic testing will increase' as genetic technologies develop. Indeed, research and experience clearly reveal a tendency to assume the desirability of preventing the birth of children with certain conditions and thus attribute, by implication, a negative value, an automatic tragic cast, to people living with those conditions. Were other groups facing oppression and stigma – people from particular ethnic groups, gay men and lesbians – automatically categorized as lives so blighted as not to be worth living, this would clearly be labelled as racism or homophobia. There was outrage a few years ago at the prospect of using a 'gay gene' for selective termination purposes, despite the fact that what was forecast was further reproductive 'choice'.

To be able to make their own decisions without external pressure, parents need to know not only how the genetic condition of the fetus may affect the life of the person to be born, but also that the society in which they and the child will live is committed to providing them with help and support. Only if prospective parents are assured that all people, however disabled, have a serious chance of receiving respect and support can they make a decision on the basis of their own values. We are a long way from there yet.

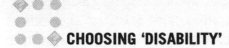

CHOOSING 'DISABILITY'

For people with achondroplasia (colloquially known as dwarfism) it may be difficult to carry and to care for and harder to achieve a pregnancy with an average-sized baby or toddler. A deaf couple may be as anxious as a non-deaf couple faced with a deaf child about not sharing a first language. Is this about 'health'? Or are these parents seeking to make 'consumer' decisions just like those parents who campaign to be allowed to clone or to select on the basis of sex or other attributes? Is being deaf harmful? Undoubtedly, if someone were deafened through negligence, compensation would be sought for them. However, many people who are born deaf, particularly where they have had the advantage of learning and using sign language from an early age, regard themselves as a cultural and linguistic minority, not as in any way 'disabled' or damaged.

From regarding a deaf child born to deaf parents as something to celebrate, it is a short step to considering the intentional abortion of 'deaf' fetuses or the rejecting of 'deaf' embryos as a form of genocide; something that is harmful at the level of society in the same way as sex selective terminations of pregnancy. In other words, individual acts of ending pregnancies are part of a wider pattern of negativity or aggression against one sex or against groups with another characteristic – in this case deafness. Genocide is a particularly emotive term when it comes to deafness, as people born deaf have a history of being discouraged from using sign language – children's hands slapped down – leaving them isolated from one another in an attempt to obliterate language and culture. The threat here is of a dwindling community to 'continue the line'.

The, to many, extraordinary preference of a few deaf people for aborting a fetus because it is not deaf, or selecting for deafness by preimplantation genetic diagnosis, seems monstrous, whereas aborting a fetus because it would have Down's Syndrome, spina bifida or be born to a mother doing her 'A' levels does not. The fetus has been personalized. It has a particular characteristic – of non-deafness – and for this it will be 'killed'. If you share a feeling of outrage about this possibility, it may perhaps bring you a step closer to understanding why proud and happy deaf and disabled people, facing daily discrimination, view pre-natal selection as discriminatory. The deaf are a cohesive community, with a rich cultural heritage and a growing body of drama, poetry and other artistic work. As Oliver Sacks points out in his book *Seeing Voices: A Journey into the World of the Deaf*: 'Sign is the equal of speech, lending itself equally to the rigorous and the poetic – to philosophical analysis or to making love – indeed, with an ease that is sometimes greater than that of speech.'

However, Adrienne Asch, herself disabled, rejects the view that preimplantation genetic diagnosis, if it is to become widely available, could be used to select to include traits such as deafness. Asch's argument is based on her stance on the pre-natal *exclusion* of particular characteristics: the part is once again being mistaken for the whole. The single characteristic is being raised to the status of only determinant in the potential for a rich and positive life.

◈◉◉
◉◉◉ WOMEN'S RIGHTS,
◉◉◈ DISABILITY RIGHTS

We are most of us ambivalent in our feelings about ending a life before birth, bringing to it our own religious or ethical beliefs, a political perspective and personal experiences. The law in Great Britain regarding abortion, for example, is a flawed compromise pleasing neither those who believe in women's absolute right to autonomy over whether and when they have children or those who believe that abortion is murder. Doctors may grant an abortion on the grounds of women's welfare, the welfare of any existing children and on grounds of the likelihood of 'serious handicap'. The latter criterion allows for termination beyond the usual 24-week limit. Counter-pressures bubble beneath the surface. We do not have abortion on demand, where the criterion would be only a woman or a couple making decisions about her or their own future. The 'right' to abortion is granted and limited by medical authority.

In outlining the limited circumstances of legal abortion and specifying 'serious handicap', a message is conveyed that abortion is the right thing to do. It is, perhaps, understandable to try to prevent women who terminate a wanted pregnancy because it may be affected by impairment from feeling guilty. They should not do so. In my view, no one should be forced to continue any 'unviable' (in terms of gestation) pregnancy that they do not want. Women make difficult choices and this should be no one's business but theirs and perhaps their partners. However, while women in these circumstances may be vulnerable and need support to overcome feelings of guilt, in restricting abortion but 'allowing' it on grounds of impairment, a woman's 'choice' to terminate is, in media parlance, 'spun' – not as a personal decision about the course of her own life, but as an act of valour benefiting her not-to-be-born fetus.

This is frustrating to many disabled people engaged in struggles for social and political change. All lives are blighted by circumstances beyond our control: contracting illness or disease, failed relationships and the deaths of loved ones. All of us bring our different personalities and capacities to the trials and traumas of life and, perhaps surprisingly, snatch moments of pleasure and satisfaction from life. Disabled people do this too. They laugh, love, cry and generally do all the mundane, clichéd things like anyone else. Yet our culture singles out those who differ substantially from the average and imposes a view of their lives as of abject tragedy. In addition, in turning away from the inevitable frailties of human life, most societies have shut disabled people out – of transport, of employment, of communication systems. In attempting to deny the existence and inevitability for most of us of illness, impairment and death, you could say that society turns away, attempts to forget, tries to banish to the margins. Hence the inaccessible pub or the school that doesn't want you because you are blind.

What is frustrating for many disabled people is the way the perception – 'disabled people lead miserable lives' – becomes the reality *but not because*, or *not only because*, of our impairments. This is the central reason why the British disability movement, and similar movements in other parts of the world, feel this issue of selection so intensely.

MAKING A CHOICE: POLICY RECOMMENDATIONS

This essay explores the 'disability equality perspective' on the subject of genetic selection. I have indicated that, while there is some consensus and a number of public statements from disability organizations on these issues, there are also different views and continuing debate. These are often painful, personal and difficult issues as well as issues of public policy. As I argued here, each of us brings our own particular experiences and beliefs to the table. So, in turning to concrete recommendations, I will give you just one disability perspective – my own.

I write as a disabled woman, with at least one known 'genetic condition', which affects my spine and is shared with my father and my sister. My own form of 'disability oppression', felt acutely in my teens and twenties, stemmed directly from the possibility of 'passing it on' – of failing my child as a parent and of being genetically tainted. I do not feel these things today. While I would not wish specifically to ensure a child of mine shared this particular characteristic, I would not regard it as inimical to life. This viewpoint is shared by many disabled people with conditions that have far more profound an impact on their lives and life expectancy than mine.

I also write as a woman who believes very strongly in women's right to self-determination and autonomy and that women's decisions about reproduction at the 'pre-viable' stage are a matter only for their own conscience. However, I also believe that there is a balance between individual and collective rights and that concerns of equality have a bearing and are affected by individual decisions. In relation to current policy, I would like to see greater freedom within more clearly defined limits, which may sound all too paradoxical!

First, I believe that there should be a common time limit for all terminations of pregnancy. Wherever in the process of gestation we choose to accord recognition of independent status to the fetus, broadly accepted to be around the time at which it might be capable of life outside its mother's body, albeit with medical support, that should be common to all fetuses: equality before the law. To deviate from this is to espouse the view that lives vary in value and rights.

Second, I would like to see major change in the provision of ante-natal services, with renewed efforts to achieve impartiality, greater access to information about what the lives of disabled people are and can be like, rather than a sole concentration on the medical aspects of people's lives. Disabled people have a vital role in preparing materials that can speak directly to parents.

Third, there needs to be far greater support for parents who choose knowingly to continue a pregnancy where the child will be disabled. This should be viewed as a positive act of love for the child to be and a confirmation of a parent's acceptance of their parenting role, whatever the individual characteristics or circumstances of their child.

Fourth, the previous point need not imply that it is morally wrong for women or couples to make reproductive decisions, including termination of pregnancy, at a stage prior to when a fetus might be capable of being born alive. However, the emphasis should be on that woman or couple making a decision based on what she or they want for her or their own future and family, not based on a judgement that a life is not worth living. For this to be possible, however, a more liberal approach to abortion would be required.

Fifth, preimplantation genetic diagnosis, in my view, should never be used to choose 'desirable' characteristics. It risks profoundly eugenic outcomes. It provides welcome possibilities to some individuals or couples who are unable to achieve a viable pregnancy. It provides the possibility of avoiding some conditions that result in an early death. Again, for pragmatic reasons, I believe this should be available in limited circumstances for conditions of this type, not because lives that are short or that contain pain or distress are less valid or that children and adults facing these things are incapable of positive experiences.

Finally, I would echo remarks of Tom Shakespeare's: that we share 98 per cent of our genetic material with chimpanzees and 51 per cent of it with yeast. Genes do not tell us the meaning of life. They do not provide the blueprint for life. We are more than our genes. Being a good parent is surely not about enhancing our children but about enhancing our children's lives through making them feel loved, accepted and wanted.

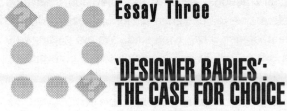

'DESIGNER BABIES': THE CASE FOR CHOICE

Juliet Tizzard

In August 2000 a baby named Adam was born to Jack and Lisa Nash, a young couple from Colorado in the USA. Adam looked like a perfectly normal baby – and he was. But his conception was brought about in a way that made medical history. Adam was conceived by means of preimplantation genetic diagnosis, performed so that a child would be born free from Fanconi's anaemia, a disease affecting the Nash's six-year-old daughter, Molly. But the novelty was in another test performed on the batch of embryos from which Adam emerged. The embryos were tested for Fanconi's anaemia and then tested for their tissue type. Those free from the disease and with the same tissue type as Molly were transferred to Lisa Nash's womb. The result was Adam.

This was the first time that PGD had been used not only to avoid a particular genetic disease, but also to provide an opportunity for donor tissue matching. Thus, Mr and Mrs Nash were able to have a child, knowing from the beginning of the pregnancy that their baby would not suffer in the same way that their daughter Molly had. Better, the birth of their new baby brought with it hope that Molly could be treated and her life could be saved. For the Nashes, PGD offered the only hope of protecting the health and well-being of both their children.

Not every one greeted Adam's birth with as much delight as his parents and sister. Within hours of the story breaking, a host of journalists, commentators and experts stepped forward to pass judgement on the Nash's actions. Articles and television interviews were littered with references to 'designer babies'. Speaking to the BBC, anti-genetics campaigner David King said: 'We are getting into a designer babies era, what I would call a eugenics area... to picking and choosing our children' (4 October 2000).

But while the *Daily Mail* hailed Adam Nash as the 'first true designer baby', most commentators went no further than to suggest that Adam's birth was the thin end of the wedge. 'This could be the start of a slippery slope,' observed philosopher Jonathan Glover (*Independent*, 4 October 2000). Few people actually objected to the Nash's specific use of PGD. Instead, most were concerned about what other uses it might lead to. In common with much media debate around PGD and 'designer babies', the prospect of the 'slippery slope', from the current use of PGD, to a worrysome future, was raised.

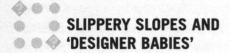

SLIPPERY SLOPES AND 'DESIGNER BABIES'

Very few commentators felt able to criticize Jack and Lisa Nash for seeking to protect the health of their children. Only those who oppose anything which involves the destruction of human embryos felt compelled to object without reservation. 'In essence it is about people being killed to get the child you want,' said Kevin Male on behalf of the anti-abortion group, Life. Others were less concerned with this specific use of PGD and more worried about where this might lead in the future. Would PGD for Fanconi's anaemia and tissue typing encourage more trivial uses of the technology in years to come?

This concern about a slippery slope to 'designer babies' was reiterated in a more recent PGD case. An unnamed couple requested PGD to select out Li-Fraumeni Syndrome, an inherited predisposition to many forms of cancer caused by a mutation in a tumour-suppressing gene called P53. American bioethicist Art Caplan raised similar concerns about this case to those which had been raised at the time of Adam Nash's birth: 'While a test to prevent a high risk of a fatal cancer makes ethical sense, what will happen when testing extends to height, eye color, muscular strength, hair color and other traits that are highly determined by our genes?' (*MSNBC*, 8 June 2001).

The media discussion around these and other PGD cases demonstrates a fear that the technique might soon be used for the selection of characteristics, rather than to screen out life-threatening diseases. But is this fear legimate? Many of the characteristics mentioned by Caplan are caused largely by genetic factors. But many are caused by a number of genes, interacting with one another and, in some instances, with non-genetic factors such as diet and exercise. When the genetic basis of such characteristics is better understood, it might one day be possible to screen for them at the embryo stage, assuming that there were any demand for such use of the technology. But until that time, the reasons for which PGD is performed are rather more mundane.

THE CURRENT REALITY OF PGD

In the United Kingdom, there are just five clinics which have a licence to provide preimplantation genetic diagnosis to patients. In the 12 years of its availability, the number of babies born as a result of PGD – performed for a handful of rare, serious diseases – has not gone beyond a few hundred. Because it involves *in vitro* fertilization (IVF), PGD is a costly exercise rarely provided for on the National Health Service. Besides often feeling physically – and emotionally – drained after having going through PGD, couples who do use PGD often find themselves thousands of pounds poorer too. And if the odds have gone against them (as it does in 70 per cent of cases) they will also find themselves without a baby to show for it.

None of this is to say that PGD is not worth it for the people who undergo it – even for those who do not succeed in their quest to have a healthy child. It is simply to demonstrate that the picture of PGD that is often painted in the media today is woefully far from reality. 'Designer babies' are simply not a feature of PGD at the current time. Instead, the treatment is characterized by waiting, hoping, paying rather a lot of money and, more often than not, failing.

This skewed picture of PGD, painted by the discussion around 'designer babies', is clearly unfortunate and no doubt frustrating for those involved, but does it really matter that much? Perhaps focusing upon what might happen in the future is a way of ensuring against complacency, of alerting us to problems before they arise. Unfortunately, the outcome of this concern about future abuses is doing more harm than good.

◆◦◦
◦ ◦ WHY THE 'DESIGNER BABIES' DEBATE
◦ ◦◆ IS HARMFUL

We have seen how today's debate about 'designer babies' is future focused. But does this really matter? Thinking ahead about what might happen in the future seems pretty harmless. It could even be considered a rather sensible approach. But a focus on the future rather than the present is often counter-productive and can even do more harm than good. It can lead to overregulation for current requirements, making access to services more restricted than it need be. It trivializes current use of the technology by making an association with 'designer babies' and fails to address current problems with *limited* service provision. Finally, a focus on future possible abuses of reproductive and genetic technologies leads ultimately to reproductive choice being undermined.

OVERREGULATION

Commentators often voice concern about 'things getting out of control'. But these concerns do not simply represent a vague worry about unrestrained reproductive choice. With warnings of slippery slopes come very real demands for constraint and control, over and above existing regulations.

PGD is regulated by the Human Fertilisation and Embryology Act passed in 1990. But precisely how and which PGD services are made available to the public is a matter for the judgement of the Human Fertilisation and Embryology Authority (HFEA), a watchdog established by the Act. At present, the HFEA requires that each new disease that PGD clinics wish to test for must be subject to a specific licence. This means that not only must the test be prepared in the laboratory (which can take some months) but a new licence application process must be entered into each time a test for a new disease is performed. This can lead to a long wait on the part of the patient, who is no doubt anxious to embark upon treatment.

It is not clear why this individualized approach to PGD regulation is necessary. PGD clinics are already subject to a licence to perform IVF treatment, a licence which requires the clinic to collect data on treatment cycles and report them to the HFEA; to be subject to annual on-site inspections; to write and adhere to laboratory, clinic and ethical protocols; and to act in a way which promotes the welfare of a child who might be born as a result of treatment. Clinics also have to secure a licence to practise PGD itself. This is granted when the HFEA is satisfied that embryologists can perform a single-cell biopsy of an embryo and that the clinic has established a system of collaboration between an assisted conception team, genetic counsellors and genetics laboratory staff. Adding to this regulation and monitoring by requiring permission for each genetic disease testing seems an unnecessary burden on the clinic and the patient.

Like many watchdogs, the HFEA is keen to be seen to be controlling reproductive medicine very closely. A debate about PGD where constant calls for legal controls are made can only encourage the HFEA to regulate further, leading to a situation where rules are laid down not in response to the needs of patients, but in order to meet a perceived public demand for limits. This is no way to regulate, and can only mean that the question of meeting the needs of the people who really matter – the patients – is rarely addressed.

TRIVIALIZING CURRENT USE

An unhealthy focus on 'designer babies' also means that the reasons for which couples currently request PGD are trivialized. The small number of couples who come forward for PGD usually do so after all other options have failed them. They may have had an affected child or perhaps one or more terminations of pregnancy or, in the case of a condition like Huntington's disease, they may have witnessed the suffering and death of family members. People request this treatment because they simply cannot leave reproduction to chance any more. The normal delights of pregnancy – wondering how the genetic die has rolled for their prospective child – are rarely shared by those at risk of having a child with a genetic disease. They have lost the reproductive confidence that everyone else takes for granted.

Talking about these perfectly legitimate reasons for requesting PGD in the same breath as using the technique to choose the eye colour or physique of one's offspring makes an erroneous association between the two. It tars PGD patients of today with the same brush as those who might wish to 'design' their children in the future.

Such concentration on PGD for the selection of particular characteristics also serves to distract us from some of the real problems that current patients face. IVF treatment (an integral part of PGD) is expensive, invasive and often emotionally draining. Each cycle of treatment can cost up to £3,000 in the United Kingdom (and much more in the United States), a financial burden which usually falls on the patient because only 10 per cent of IVF treatment is provided by the National Health Service. And because each cycle has around a 30 per cent success rate, patients tend to need two or more treatments in order to conceive. The IVF cycle involves an intense drug regime – with a number of side-effects – and an invasive procedure to collect the matured eggs for fertilization. None of this is to say that IVF should not be available or is not worth undergoing, even for those who do not succeed. But for couples at risk of having a child with a genetic disease – couples who do not usually *need* fertility treatment – PGD is no picnic, physically or psychologically.

The range of PGD services available in the United Kingdom is extremely limited. More than a decade after its inception, the technique is performed for just a handful of genetic disorders and a few inherited cancers in five UK clinics. The conditions are individually rare, often fatal (or seriously debilitating) and the offspring have a high chance of inheriting them (usually one in two or one in four). Although little research has been carried out on couples undergoing PGD treatment, the limited services that are currently available in the United Kingdom are valued enormously by patients. Many have had an affected child (and perhaps seen him or her die at an early age) or a number of terminations of pregnancy. Some have a personal objection to abortion and think of PGD as the only acceptable option besides leaving things to chance. Regardless of the reasons for requesting it, PGD offers an option to those people who feel that they have run out of alternatives.

The real concern about PGD should be how limited it is. In the United Kingdom, there are a small number of diseases that can be tested for and only a few centres in which to receive treatment. Yet, these real limitations are rarely discussed because they are eclipsed by overblown worries about non-medical uses and 'designer babies'.

UNDERMINING CHOICE

The final disadvantage of focusing too much on possible future abuses of PGD technology is that it undermines choice. In all the talk of 'designer babies', the idea that reproductive choice is a good thing has been eroded. Instead, choice has become associated with selfishness, indulgence and even harm. Reproductive choice is an important liberty which should be enjoyed by every member of society. As autonomous adults, we ought to be allowed to make decisions about our personal lives according to our own needs and desires. Indeed, our ability to do so is something we take for granted. Most people would be outraged by the suggestion that anyone other than they should set down rules about, or intervene in, the conduct of their sex life for example. In the case of reproduction, parents take the major burden of responsibility for their children, for identifying and protecting their best interests. In order to do this best, the choice about when, where and how those children are conceived and born must be the preserve of the parents.

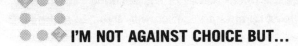

I'M NOT AGAINST CHOICE BUT...

Nowadays, few people would disagree entirely with the notion that reproductive choice matters. But support for individuals exercising choice is often limited or inconsistent. People often say that they are all in favour of women (and their partners) having reproductive choice, but add that it should not be unlimited choice or that it should be restrained in some circumstances. So, what are the arguments put forward to justify limits to personal choice? Two concerns about personal choice currently have a high profile, both of which argue that choice is not always benign; it often affects, even harms, other people. Those people, it is claimed, are either disabled people in the population or the children who are born as a result of exercising personal choice.

ATTITUDES TOWARDS DISABLED PEOPLE

Many of those involved in promoting the interests of disabled people are concerned that preimplantation and pre-natal diagnosis – both the provision of services and the choice to use those services – have negative effects on disabled people. One argument made is that the choice to have, or not to have, a disabled child is not a real choice. This is because, it is claimed, society imposes beliefs on us that tend us towards one decision: namely, to avoid the birth of a disabled child.

Following this logic however, all choices people make become suspect. No choice is made outside the influences of society. For example, all prospective parents make decisions about reproduction based on the realities of life: the cost of childcare or of housing, whether friends and family have children or whether they, as parents, are able to emotionally provide for their children. While most of these constraints are changeable (more money or social support could help lessen their impact), most parents just get on with trying to make the best possible environment for their children. Similar practical considerations are made by prospective parents of a disabled child. But, in addition, they might need to think about what medical or social services are or are not available to help with their child, where he or she will go to school, what employment prospects they have and whether they will be able to lead an independent adult life. Advocates of the social model of disability argue that because of this, if the choice is made not to have a child with a disability, the choice is suspect. The inadequacy of services for disabled people means that a real choice has not been made, since if services were improved, the choice made may be different. How valid is this argument?

Poor social services, few employment opportunities and a lack of adequate housing and support are certainly all problematic constraints for disabled people today – and they no doubt have some bearing on reproductive decision making. But that is not to say that, if these pressures were eliminated, the choice between having a disabled child or not having a disabled child would be completely equivalent. Regardless of how much services improve, it is likely that for many prospective parents, the prospect of having a disabled child is not one that they consider best for them.

One reason for this is that there is a reality associated with caring for a disabled child caused by the condition itself. With a condition such as cystic fibrosis (the most common inherited condition in the UK), the child's health is often at risk and many hospital visits are required in early life. In cases of mental impairment, the child may not be able to enjoy life to the same fullness that able bodied children are. A child with Down's Syndrome will probably (depending upon the severity of the condition) never become a fully independent adult, able to drive a car or live alone or have a family or live until 85. These are not necessarily reasons not to have a child with a disability, but they are real considerations that it is perfectly legitimate for parents to take into consideration when faced with a positive pre-natal test result.

Another criticism made of pre-natal diagnosis is that its very existence implies a negative attitude towards existing disabled people. The use of services by prospective parents, it is claimed, furthers the notion that people with disabilities are somehow less valuable or worthwhile as people, than those without disabilities and is therefore damaging. So does the choice to screen pre-natally damage the lives of disabled people? When a prospective parent is faced with a choice about whether to proceed with a pregnancy or to terminate it, does that choice 'say' anything about disabled people in general?

Some parents, particularly those who already have a disabled child, might feel that their choice to terminate an affected fetus has an impact beyond that pregnancy. But most parents in this situation are able to separate their existing child from the condition from which they suffer. They love and care for that child while not wanting their next child to suffer from the same condition. However, by using genetic screening to avoid a particular disease or disability, parents are making a personal, not a social, choice.

And so, a couple's decision – whether to continue a pregnancy or to end it – is one that is best for them, not one which they would wish to be generalized across society. A comparable illustration of this is the case of older women. A significant proportion of women who have abortions for non-medical reasons are those who have already completed their family and get pregnant accidentally some years after the birth of their youngest child. If a woman in this position chooses to have an abortion, she is not saying that older women should not have children; she is simply saying that having another child is not right for her, her partner and her existing children.

If an individual choice to avoid the birth of a disabled child does not have a negative effect on disabled people, what about the existence of screening services themselves? Some have argued that the mere existence of services which seek to identify affected embryos or fetuses assumes that avoiding the birth of a disabled or sick child is a desirable thing to do. Just as screening for breast cancer assumes that avoiding or curing breast cancer is a good thing, are genetic screening services based upon the assumption that avoiding genetic disease is also a good thing?

It is clear that screening for genetic disease and chromosomal abnormality was not established simply to enhance reproductive choice, although that has been an effect. Pre-natal diagnosis services were established to help parents at risk of having a child with an inherited disease avoid having a child with that disease. Studies show that many of these couples, before the introduction of pre-natal diagnosis, had decided to forego having children for precisely this reason. The new services enabled them to rediscover a sense of confidence about having children that they had long since lost.

Another consideration in the provision of pre-natal and preimplantation screening services is economic. Healthcare economists know that screening and associated obstetric services are, in the long run, cheaper than the health and social care services required to help a disabled child and adult through life. This is an unpleasant reality of healthcare provision, but it is one which cannot be ignored.

And so, the existence of pre-natal and preimplantation genetic diagnostic services does presuppose that the avoidance of genetic disease in children is a desirable goal, both medically and economically. But this does not mean that children or adults with a genetic disease should never have been born. Neither does it mean that parents should be encouraged to use screening services to avoid the birth of an affected child. Just as a woman with a breast cancer diagnosis as a result of screening is not obliged to accept whatever treatment is offered to her, a woman with a diagnosis of fetal abnormality is not obliged to terminate her pregnancy. In fact, the latter woman is more likely to be treated sympathetically in her refusal of an abortion than is the woman refusing breast cancer treatment. Women or couples offered pre-natal screening have every right to refuse tests or to refuse a termination of pregnancy when a test reveals an abnormality. Like the decision to have a test or end a pregnancy, this decision should be respected and supported by health practitioners and society at large.

While genetic screening services might be offered with a particular use in mind, using those services for that particular use is by no means obligatory. The services are not based on eugenic assumptions, but on the assumption that, all things being equal, it is better that children are born healthy, rather than sick or disabled. However, those that *are* born sick or disabled (either through choice or misfortune) should be cared and provided for like any other child.

CHILDREN AS PRODUCTS

Some commentators, concerned about reproductive choice, fear that those who exercise it will ultimately be disappointed by their children. As choice is extended, they argue, parents will develop a 'consumerist' attitude towards their children, thus fundamentally changing the relationship between parent and child. But what do they mean by this? To be a consumer is to buy a product one desires, to use it and to throw it away when it has served its purpose. Does this relationship apply to parent and child, as it does to consumer and product?

It is difficult to measure whether parents have a more 'consumerist' attitude towards their children today, largely because those who make this accusation rarely back it up with proof of its existence. But let's assume that there might be ways of telling whether reproductive choice leads to parents having a consumerist attitude towards their children. If reproductive consumerism is about using and then discarding children (just as we use and discard products), then we might expect to find more mistreated and, ultimately, abandoned children around today. Are more children being taken into care because their parents mistreat or no longer want them? No, they are not.

If enhanced reproductive choice means that parents have higher expectations of their children, then we might expect to find more children alive today who feel unable to live up to parental hopes for them (because no child can surely live up to such expectations). Those parents who might be considered as having exercised the most choice in relation to their children are those who have used assisted reproduction (IVF and associated techniques) to conceive. But psychological research studies show that children born of assisted reproductive techniques (ART) fare just as well in their psychological development and in the relationship with their parents as children who were conceived naturally. ART parents, people who arguably have the highest expectations of their children by virtue of having gone through so much to have them, show no signs of rearing psychologically damaged offspring. And ART children are certainly not more likely to end up in care because of mistreatment or lack of love.

The truth is that people who go through so much to have a child, either because of infertility or because they wish to avoid passing down a genetic disease, show no signs of treating their offspring as products. Choice in reproduction and in the marketplace are not the same thing, nor should they be considered as such. Those who take advantage of the choice offered by reproductive technologies want, love and nurture their children just as much as those who are able to leave reproduction to chance.

◆●●
●　●
●　●◆ **CONCLUSION:**
FOR OR AGAINST CHOICE

In the debate around preimplantation and pre-natal testing, there are only two possible positions to take. Either one is in favour of women or couples making their own reproductive decisions or one is not. It is simply not a sustainable argument to say 'I'm in favour of choice, but...'.

Some oppose choice because of anti-abortion concerns. For them, women's choice is always a problem because it opens up the possibility of destroying embryonic or fetal life which they consider sacrosanct. This approach is internally consistent, but it is an argument which also opposes all reproductive technologies, including some methods of contraception, which involve loss of embryos. The case made by others, who are not anti-abortion, but who argue that choice ought to be constrained are harder to appreciate. Without good justification for limits to reproductive choice, such opponents seem to rely more upon personal prejudice than on sound principle.

To say that choice ought to be limited to ensure against abuse is not to say that no choice should be exercised at all. It is to say that the choice ought to be given to someone other than the women or couple involved. If Parliament decides that women who, for instance, discover that their fetus is suffering from Down's Syndrome are not allowed an abortion, the decision has not been magicked away. It has already been made by politicians on their behalf.

The best way to ensure against abuse is to allow people seeking PGD to make their own choice about their own children, just as everyone else is allowed to do. People want to exercise reproductive choice for different reasons: perhaps because of difficult circumstances or because of a legitimate desire to maximize the health of their children. What is worrying is not unrestrained choice, but the participation of third parties in that decision-making process: doctors, politicians, lawyers or even pressure groups. Allowing third parties to make reproductive decisions on behalf of women and couples without their permission is more of a threat to society than the mythical 'designer baby' ever could be.

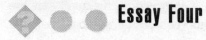

Essay Four

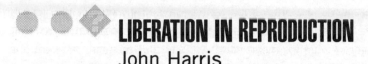

LIBERATION IN REPRODUCTION
John Harris

What if any, constraints or limitations should there be on the use of assisted reproductive technologies (ART)? How far should people be free to choose not only their broad reproductive path but also its finer byways? That is, not only choose how and when and why to reproduce, but also to have control of other features of reproduction including phenotypic traits of children (features like hair, eye and skin colour, general physique, intelligence or sporting ability and the like) that are susceptible to technological or genetic manipulation.

HOW MIGHT INTERVENTIONS IN REPRODUCTION BE JUSTIFIED?

Let's start by asking when interventions in the reproductive process might be legitimate and, since such interventions are an instance of medical interventions more generally, we must start with a prior question: When is the use of technology for medical and therapeutic purposes morally justified? A first and obvious answer is that it is justified when it will do good and where any harmful side-effects are small compared with the good and where it will not violate anyone's rights. So, the good achieved, the importance of that good and the fact that it is desired by those whom it benefits or (where patients cannot request or consent to its use) is in their best interests are the important factors. The importance of medical interventions is proportional to the magnitude of the good that they will do and the use of the interventions will be ethical if they will do the good that the patients want or when patients cannot request interventions, their use will be ethical if it does good and is in the patient's best interests.

Medical 'goods' are often important because they protect life, lessen pain or suffering, restore mobility and so on. But note that there is an ambiguity in what we mean when we say that medical interventions are justified by the good that they do. There is ambiguity between the questions of whether the deployment of public resources for the achievement of the particular good, on the one hand, is justified and whether individuals are justified in accessing or others are justified in offering treatments, on the other. The use of public resources may be justified if interventions do a good that ought to be done, although pressure on resources will always influence what is actually funded. But the individuals will be justified in using and others justified in providing treatments or interventions if they do no harm, or no significant harm, even if there are no moral imperatives for doing that harmless or marginally harmful thing.

Most elective medical procedures, including male circumcision or breast enhancements would be justifiable in this way. If the surgery is necessary to prevent or mitigate suffering then it will be justified both to do it and to spend public resources on it. But if it is purely a matter of personal preference – I'd like larger breasts or a modified penis, but my life is not made intolerable by my natural endowments – then interventions, while not required by morality and while not in the public interest, are not wrongful in any way. However, if the individual wants an intervention that although only mildly harmful to her is immoral for independent reasons, the case is different. Having a racist slogan indelibly burnt into one's forehead would be an example of this kind, in that it constitutes incitement to racial hatred, is against the public interest and is arguably harmful or a danger to others.

The provision of services which require technology, even medical technology is morally neutral, aside that is from the consequences (including the costs) of providing them. There is nothing special about 'medical' technology and it shares the justifications of the practice of medicine more generally. Shorn of those general justifications it requires its own. And here the question of the burden of proof arises. Who has to justify what?

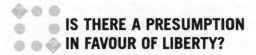

IS THERE A PRESUMPTION IN FAVOUR OF LIBERTY?

In most democracies (but not all) there is a presumption in favour of liberty. Such a presumption means that the burden of justifying their actions falls on those who would deny liberty not on those who would exercise it. If this is right, the presumption must be in favour of the liberty to access ART unless good and sufficient reasons can be shown against so doing. But suppose this presumption is not accepted. Can anything else be said about the liberty to access ART which might support such a presumption?

REPRODUCTIVE LIBERTY

When people express their choices about procreation they are claiming an ancient, if only recently firmly established, example of what may be termed a 'fundamental right'. This right or entitlement is found in all the principal conventions or declarations of human rights. Sometimes it is expressed as the right to marry and found a family, sometimes as the right to privacy and to respect for family life (see the United Nations Universal Declaration of Human Rights, Article 16 1978, the European Convention on Human Rights, Article 8 and Article 12, 1953 and the International Covenant of Civil and Political Rights, Article 23, 1976). This right or entitlement is often discussed in terms of 'reproductive liberty' or 'procreative autonomy'.

The right or entitlement to reproductive liberty has a number of different sources and justifications. Some see it as derived from the right to reproduce *per se*, others as derivative of other important rights or freedoms (see for example my *Wonderwoman & Superman: The Ethics of Human Biotechnology*, Oxford University Press, 1992 and, for a more explicit, elegant defence John A. Robertson, *Children of Choice*, Princeton University Press, 1994 and Ronald Dworkin, *Life's Dominion*, HarperCollins, 1993). Certainly, there is no widespread agreement as to the nature and scope of this right; however, it is clear that it must apply to more than conventional sexual reproduction and that it includes a range of the values and liberties which normal sexual reproduction embodies or subserves. For example, John Robertson outlining his understanding of this right suggests:

> The moral right to reproduce is respected because of the centrality of reproduction to personal identity, meaning and dignity. This importance makes the liberty to procreate an important moral right, both for an ethic of individual autonomy and for the ethics of community or family that view the purpose of marriage and sexual union as the reproduction and rearing of offspring. Because of this importance the right to reproduce is widely recognised as a prima facie moral right that cannot be limited except for very good reason.
>
> *Children of Choice*, Princeton University Press, 1994

Ronald Dworkin has defined reproductive liberty or procreative autonomy as 'a right to control their own role in procreation unless the state has a compelling reason for denying them that control':

> The right of procreative autonomy has an important place... in Western political culture more generally. The most important feature of that culture is a belief in individual human dignity:

that people have the moral right – and the moral responsibility – to confront the most fundamental questions about the meaning and value of their own lives for themselves, answering to their own consciences and convictions... The principle of procreative autonomy, in a broad sense, is embedded in any genuinely democratic culture.

Life's Dominion, HarperCollins 1993

Arguably Dworkin's and Robertson's accounts both centre on what I believe to be the key idea, namely respect for autonomy and for the values which underlie the importance attached to procreation. These values see procreation and founding a family as involving the freedom to choose one's own lifestyle and express, through actions as well as through words, the deeply held beliefs and the morality which families share and seek to pass on to future generations.

Given that the freedom to pass on one's genes is widely perceived to be an important value, it is natural to see this freedom as a plausible dimension of reproductive liberty, not least because so many people and agencies have been attracted by the idea of the special nature of genes and have linked the procreative imperative to the genetic imperative. Whether or not this suggestion is ultimately persuasive, it is surely not possible to dismiss the choices about reproduction and access to the relevant technologies which constitute the point of claiming reproductive liberty as a simple and idle exercise of preference. Reproductive choices, whether or not they prove to be protected by a right to procreative liberty or autonomy, have without doubt a claim to be taken seriously as moral claims. As such they may not simply be dismissed wherever and whenever a voting majority can be assembled against them. Those who seek to deny the moral claims of others (as opposed, possibly, to the exercise of their idle preferences) must show good and sufficient cause.

● ● ●
● ● IS THERE JUSTIFICATION FOR DENYING ACCESS
● ● ◆ TO ARTIFICIAL REPRODUCTIVE TECHNOLOGY?

If we can identify interventions or their consequences that would be morally problematic *of themselves* we might know which traits it would be morally problematic to produce deliberately. The answer seems to be only those traits which would be harmful to the individual produced or harmful to others. Thus it would not be a morally problematic event if a boy rather than a girl were produced (or vice versa), and it would not be morally problematic if a child with a particular skin colour, hair colour, eye colour, or a range of useful abilities – sporting prowess, musical talent, intelligence and so on – were to be born or created. It could not be said that children with any of these features would be born in a harmed condition or at any disadvantage whatsoever, and neither would it be plausible to claim that they would be in any way harmful or dangerous to others. No one has a reason to bemoan the birth of a child with any of these features or characteristics, neither would a child with such features have any ground for complaint to find him/herself a bonny, bouncing, blue-eyed, musically talented boy or a handsome, lithe, brown-eyed girl who is brilliant at football.

By the same token, we know very well that to choose to bring a child with disabilities into being is morally problematic and a child born permanently lame, deaf, blind or with short life expectancy, would surely have grounds for complaint if any of these characteristics had been deliberately chosen by its parents or indeed anyone else. Why then do some people feel that designing children to be healthy, talented or to possess one harmless or beneficial feature rather than another – skin colour hair or eye colour gender and so on – might somehow be wrong? If it is not wrong to wish for a bonny, bouncing, brown-eyed, intelligent baby girl, with athletic potential and musical ability, in virtue of what might it be wrong to use technology to play fairy godmother to oneself and grant the wish that was parent to the child?

Let's now look in more detail at individual reproductive choices that might be made and see how the principles we have identified might work.

OLDER PARENTS

Should we use ART to help older men and women including women past the natural age for the menopause to have children? Some have objected to extensions in women's ability to have children on the grounds that it is unnatural. Since the whole practice of medicine is unnatural – people naturally fall ill and die prematurely – if we were to accept an ethic which required us not to interfere with what was natural there would be little for medical practitioners and medical scientists to do. Increased risks attached to childbearing for older women have also been cited against permitting the practice. The health of the mother, while of obvious concern, is of concern principally to the mother herself. If she feels it acceptable to risk her health in pursuance of her desire to have a child, or another child, that surely is a decision for her to take. It is, of course, a risk which all mothers always take, pregnancy and childbirth being risky at whatever age they are undertaken.

It has also been claimed that post-menopausal women who are likely to be in their seventies when their children are teenagers would not be able to function adequately as parents because they may lack the energy of youth or lack physical capacity for the hard work and hard play required of parents. This is a very disturbing claim since it would debar many physically disabled parents from the right to procreate. And as for having energy in other directions, it is now commonplace for people in their sixties and seventies to be looking after their very aged parents, who may be in their eighties and nineties. This is a task which society seems to expect more and more of older people and which is, by any standards, much more demanding than looking after children.

Would the death of their parents, while the children are still quite young, be a hardship to which children should not be condemned? While there is no doubt that the loss of parents, whom one loves and on whom one depends, is distressing and problematic at any age, it is clearly likely to be the more so in children or adolescents. However, while there is some agreement in the literature, that such bereavement is a tragedy, the consensus seems to be that its harmful effects are manageable with care and support (see for example, Dora Black, 'Psychological Reactions to Life Threatening and Terminal Illness and Bereavement' in *Child Psychiatry: Modern Approaches*, M. Rutter, E. Taylor and L. Hersov (eds) Butterworth, 1994 and Rebecca Abrams, *When Parents Die*, Charles Letts, 1992). In any event, the question that must be pressed is: Does such a bereavement even in childhood or adolescence make the entire life of that child so emphatically not worth living that it would be better had they never been born or wrongful in some way to have brought them into the world? Such an outcome is surely unlikely.

DESIGNER CHILDREN

The phrase 'designer children' has clear negative connotations when used to describe children born as a result of the exercise of reproductive choice. The implication is that the parents are more concerned with fashion and pleasing themselves, than with valuing children for the children's own sake. However, normal sexual reproduction and choice of procreational partner has always had a large element of design in it. Cultures, religions and races that have encouraged their members to marry and procreate with other members of the same group are all into designer babies. It is a truism that bears repeating, that once you have the capacity to choose and the awareness of that capacity, then choice is inevitable. It is not the less an exercise of choice because the choice is exercised in a traditional or culturally approved way.

GENDER SELECTION

To address the issue of the ethics of design in procreation let's turn to a very basic element of design, namely gender. First, we need to distinguish between morally neutral and morally significant features or traits. A feature is morally neutral if its presence or absence is not morally significant. Thus it would not be *morally* better to have one colour of hair rather than another or, for that matter, to be one gender rather than another. Similarly, to have a disability or an advantage is not morally neutral. Of course, the *manner of choosing* may be morally important. We might feel that abortion was not a reasonable way of determining such things; but if, for example, a litre of orange juice taken at a particular point in pregnancy could achieve the desired outcome, I doubt if any attempt to regulate its use would succeed or ought even to be attempted. At the moment a reliable method of gender determination in humans does not exist, but it is always important to decide principles in advance of practicalities.

Objections to the idea of gender selection and the like often turn on two forms of 'slippery slope' argument. Either it is claimed that a pattern of gender preference will emerge which will constitute a sort of 'slap in the face' to the gender discriminated against, an insult and humiliation, like a piece of racist graffiti perhaps, or, it is suggested that the pattern of preference will be such as to create severe imbalance in the population of society with harmful social consequences. Plainly these are very different sorts of outcome.

We should note that a pattern of preference for one gender among those opting for gender selection would not necessarily be evidence of sexist discrimination. There might be all sorts of respectable, non-prejudicial reasons for preferring one gender to another including just having a preference for sons or daughters. A preference for producing a child of a particular gender no more necessarily implies discrimination against members of the alternate gender than does choosing to marry a co-religionist, a compatriot or someone of the same race or even class implies discrimination against other religions, nations, races or classes. Of course, if a pattern of preference in favour of one gender were to emerge it might have either or both of the effects we have noted and would certainly be cause for concern. However, it seems verging on hysteria simply to assume either that it would inevitably have these effects or that the effects would be so damaging as to warrant legislation to prevent the remotest risk of their occurring.

How can we guard against unacceptably bad effects of gender selection? One possible solution would be that a society such as the United Kingdom, of about 58 million people, could license, say, one million procedures for gender selection over a ten-year period, with options to revise the policy if severe imbalance seemed likely and was likely to prove significantly damaging to individuals or society. We could then see what patterns of selection and motivation emerged. Even if all choices went one way, the imbalance created would be relatively small before detection and a halt could be called if this seemed justifiable. I doubt that the places allocated on such a programme would be taken up (it would of course be self-financing and would not be part of the public healthcare system). It must be remembered that those who opted for gender selection would (with current technology) have to be very circumspect about their procreation and use sperm selection or preimplantation testing as the method. This would not, I guess, be wildly attractive or indeed particularly reliable. For the foreseeable future the take-up will also be limited by the availability of clinics offering the service. In any event, the way forward for a tolerant society respectful of autonomy, would surely be not to rush to legislation, but rather to license the activity with regular monitoring and see whether anything so terrible emerged that it required prohibitive legislation.

WHAT OF OTHER ELEMENTS OF DESIGN?

If there are six preimplantation embryos awaiting transfer and diagnosis reveals that three have genetic diseases and three are normal, which three should be implanted? Only those who think that it is legitimate to choose to implant the three with genetic illness believe there is no obligation to prevent preventable disease by making decisions as to whether or not babies with particular diseases should be brought into existence (I assume, contrary to fact, that all have an equal chance of successful birth). Now assume that we can tell that three are normal and three will have longer, healthier lives than the average. Is there a moral reason to prefer those with better prospects for a long healthy life? I believe so, but here the decision is tighter. In any event it seems improbable to conclude that it would be *unethical* to prefer the embryos with expectation of a longer healthier life than is normal for humans. Now assume something else, that there are another three embryos with superior intelligence genetically diagnosed prior to implantation. Again, for what it's worth, I would opt to implant the more intelligent. I can understand those who would not, but again it seems improbable that it could be *unethical* to implant those with predicted higher than normal intelligence.

Now assume that a longer, healthier more intelligent existence could be achieved by safe genetic manipulation of embryos. If it would not be unethical to capitalize on the chance 'blessings' of nature, if these could be diagnosed before implantation, what would make it unethical to confer such blessings if we had the technology to do so?

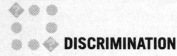

DISCRIMINATION

It is sometimes said that designing children with particular traits constitutes wrongful discrimination against people who have traits that are not chosen. It might be that the claim is that the wrongful discrimination adversely affects those who might have come into existence but for the designing strategies or the claim might be that the discrimination affects people already in existence. Not all discriminative choice is wrongful, but such choices will be wrongful if they constitute unfair discrimination. Unfair discrimination can occur in a number of ways. For our purposes it will be important to consider just three.

RELEVANT INFORMATION

Where people are disadvantaged by the decisions of others and those decisions are based on information which either is not relevant to the issue in question or is only marginally relevant to that issue, the decision can be unfair. General examples would include the relevance of racial differences used as qualifications for employment or of property qualifications for participation in the democratic process. In the case of reproductive choices decisions might be unfairly discriminatory, for example, if people believed wrongly that skin colour conferred an advantage or disadvantage. But if it were true that in countries sitting under a hole in the ozone layer, very pale skins conferred a significant additional risk of skin cancers, then Australians, for example, might have good reason to prefer to have brown-skinned children.

DEBATING MATTERS

THE MORAL OR SOCIAL CONSEQUENCES OF THE CHOICE OR DECISION

Where a decision made for relevant reasons can nonetheless be shown to be immoral or have harmful social consequences it may also constitute unfair discrimination. For example, the fact that a young woman may require maternity leave is certainly *relevant* to her utility to an organization in a particular post, but the moral wrong of excluding young women from employment or requiring them to abjure pregnancy and the harmful social consequences of discrimination on such a basis may constitute unfair discrimination. Thus a decision to select male children, when part of a pattern of such choices which seriously disadvantages members of society, might constitute unfair discrimination in this sense.

THE JUSTICE OF THE SELECTION PROCESS

Someone may, for example, be included or excluded for valid reasons but if this is part of a *process* characterized by arbitrary or inconsistent application of principles of selection the choice may be unfair. The best qualified person might in fact get the job, but if others were wrongfully disqualified from consideration, the process as a whole may be considered unfair. In the case of reproduction, if some classes of people (older parents or the poor) were denied access to reproductive technologies, while others could obtain treatment, this might constitute unfair discrimination.

CHOOSING WHO SHALL EXIST

It is sometimes said that selecting against disabilities in reproduction constitutes unfair discrimination against the disabled as a group. That this is not the case can be seen if we consider not selecting against disabilities but selecting for advantages. Suppose some embryos had a genetic condition which conferred complete immunity to many major diseases – HIV/AIDS, cancer and heart disease for example, coupled with increased longevity. We would, it seems to me, have moral reasons to prefer to implant such embryos given the opportunity of choice. But such a decision would not imply that normal people (or people who are 'normal' in 2001) have lives that are not worth living or were of poor or problematic quality. If I would prefer to confer these advantages on any future children that I may have, I am not implying that people like me, constituted as they are, have lives that are not worth living, or that are of poor quality. So existing people can have no complaints. But neither do those who might have been brought into being.

Choosing between existing people for whatever reason always involves the possibility of unfair discrimination because there will, inevitably, be people who are disadvantaged by the choice. Choosing which sorts of people to bring into existence does not adversely affect those selected against because they will never exist to be disadvantaged by the choice.

My parents were under no obligation to attempt to conceive in any particular month. If they had conceived in any month other than December 1944 I would not have existed. Not only are none of my possible siblings who have been irrevocably damaged by this choice of my parents complaining, I can assure you that had my parents chosen not to attempt to conceive that month or had their attempt – if that is what it was – been unsuccessful, you would not have heard me complain, neither would anyone else have had legitimate grounds for complaint.

Suppose *in vitro* fertilization (IVF) and preimplantation genetic diagnosis (PGD) had been available in December 1944 and 'I' had existed in a petri dish. Suppose my parents had chosen an embryo without my genetic disadvantages. Would I have had any ground for complaint? Would that have constituted discrimination against people with my genetic condition? I don't believe so. It is simply a fallacy to think that choosing between preimplantation embryos or choosing to terminate pregnancies of embryos because other embryos would have a better chance in life constitutes unfair discrimination. There is no one who is the victim of this discrimination. No one had a right to be created or to be implanted. There is no one who has an interest which is frustrated by abortion or other methods of selection.

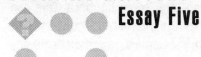

BETTER BY ACCIDENT THAN DESIGN
Josephine Quintavalle

One day every member of the human race will be beautiful and healthy and live forever and, in achieving this goal, anything is permissible. This is a dominant mantra of the western world. Man has been searching for the elixir of life since recorded time but how realistic and how morally acceptable are such dreams?

In the history of human reproduction, 25 July 1978 is a seminal date. It is the birthday of Louise Brown, the first human successfully constructed in a petri dish as opposed to conceived in a mother's body. Despite the absolute novelty of Louise's conception, the family circumstances of the Browns reflected what was at the time a reasonably normal model of family life: mother and father were in a stable marriage and Louise was their genetic child.

In the years subsequent to Louise's birth, as a consequence of laboratory techniques replacing sexual intercourse, concepts of normality have been speedily rewritten. From acceptance of what used to be known as the 'accident' of birth or for those who saw God as creator, the precious 'gift' of life, babies can now be produced for almost any person who wants one – married, single, heterosexual or homosexual. Recently the possibility of multiple genetic parents has become a reality. Mitochondrial manipulation has lead to the birth of babies with two genetic mothers and if human cloning proves feasible in the future, others will be born without genetic fathers.

The reproductive choices currently on offer seem limitless. One can buy and sell human gametes, even over the internet, post them across the world, rent surrogate wombs from catalogues, run endless quality controls on early life in the petri dish or later in the womb, put embryos on hold for years in the freezer, conceive after a partner's death and bear children long after natural menopause.

As if all these options were not sufficient, the year 2001 has brought the unveiling of the human genome, the 'book of life', with its apparent promise of unravelling the complete biological structure of human beings, thereby allowing man to rewrite himself. This massively complex annotation of our biological code, fruit of 15 years' work by thousands of international scientists, was printed out for its readers by *Science* in February 2001, on a giant poster containing the graphics of 2.9 billion genomic bases. For those of us not scientists, the human genome quickly becomes a confusion of scientific terms – chromosomes, DNA fibres, double helixes, amino acid sequences, centromeres, telomeres, proteomics, not to mention those mystifying A, T, G and Cs. What does it all mean? Basically, that scientists are looking at the body in its smallest components, with many claiming that every aspect of human identity and destiny can be traced back to how we are constructed biologically. Our present and future health patterns, neurological and behavioural expectations, will all be revealed by putting each individual genome under the microscope. A letter in *The Scotsman* (31 May 2001) referred confidently to the physiology of personality. It's all in the genes.

Or is it? A great many others reject this deterministic approach to human life, convinced that genetic analysis will never give an adequate explanation of what constitutes our humanity. Sociologist, Dr Tom Shakespeare, in a *Lancet* review, dismisses 'the hyperbole which claims that DNA is the secret of life and which reduces complex social experiences to simple molecular processes', suggesting that it is 'surely both dangerous and misplaced' to take such an approach.

What is certain is that the deciphering of the human genome has already added considerably to the field of reproductive choices. Certain genetic tests, such as those for Down's Syndrome and cystic fibrosis, are now routine in pre-natal care throughout the western world and great claims are made for the future:

> We have determined functional categories for nearly 1,000 documented disease genes, and found striking correlations between the function of the gene produce and features of disease, such as age of onset and mode of inheritance. As knowledge of disease genes grows, including those contributing to complex traits, more sophisticated analyses will be possible; their results will yield a deeper understanding of disease and an enhanced integration of medicine with biology.
>
> 'Human Disease Genes', G. Jimenez-Sanchez *et al.*,
> *Nature*, 15 February 2001

In other words, as our ability to identify defects in our genes increases, so will our ability to correct, enhance or replace the undesirable traits. We will be able to design babies.

This essay draws attention to negative aspects of these developments and argues that there are compelling reasons for rejecting the drive to make reproduction ever more technological and for restating the case for allowing nature to take its course.

◆●●
●　●　**THE MEDICAL LIMITATIONS OF**
●　●◆　**REPRODUCTIVE TECHNOLOGY**

For all the talk of 'designer' babies, 'design' is hardly an appropriate description of what is happening in assisted reproduction today. First, *in vitro* fertilization (IVF) has resulted in the ability to produce children who are not as healthy as those conceived naturally; the imperative of perfection and design is often subservient to the absolute desire for a child. The high incidence of multiple births associated with this technology has serious consequences for the health of the children produced. A technique used in male infertility, intracytoplasmic sperm injection (ICSI), where immature sperm are injected directly into the ovum, appears to increase the risk of sex chromosome abnormalities. The Italian gynaecologist, Dr Severino Antinori, at a conference in Rome in March 2001, announced plans to clone an infertile man and was blissfully unconcerned about the inevitability of replicating the father's infertility in the baby. He also shelved any concerns regarding the high levels of abnormality which have come to light in animal cloning.

Second, while many accuse those involved in assisted reproduction of having turned the baby into a designer product, they are certainly not drafting the baby from scratch. They simply expose existing embryos or fetuses in the womb to a battery of quality controls to identify 'defects' and then discard the inadequate embryo or abort the imperfect fetus.

Once it has been accepted, the baby then has to face an increasing number of medical tests, to ensure that there is no evidence of abnormality. The most widely applied tests are for Down's Syndrome and cystic fibrosis and the UK Government has pledged to make both tests universally available. At the present time around 1,800 pregnancies are terminated annually in England and Wales on the ground of fetal abnormality.

This kind of negative 'design' approach, whereby 'defective' life is simply destroyed, is also applied to early embryos. Once it became relatively easy to create human lives in the laboratory, preimplantation genetic diagnosis (PGD) soon followed. PGD may well become more sophisticated in the future but is currently a fairly crude diagnostic tool, based often on simply sexing the embryo, given that X-linked disorders are sex related, and destroying the embryos of the undesired sex. Duchenne muscular dystrophy or haemophilia, for example, only affect males, so after IVF the male embryos will be discarded and only females selected for implantation. The American Society for Reproductive Medicine claims that about 200 disorders could one day be eliminated by using gender selection, and gives a further list of 15 specific genetic diseases (either single gene or chromosomal abnormalities) which can be identified by existing technology. Sexing to avoid X-linked disorders and testing for age-related abnormalities are the most common applications of PGD worldwide and this technology was first applied in 1990 to produce two sets of twin girls whose families were at high risk of passing on a serious X-linked disorder.

Leaving to one side for the moment the big question of whether we should use a 'quality-control' approach to human life, it should be noted that no currently existing testing procedure can as yet guarantee foolproof results. The search for a particular feature (for example, a hormone level) which indicates the presence or absence of a disease depends on the acceptance of averages. These are often very difficult to establish, with considerable overlap between healthy and unhealthy measurements. It is difficult to find statistics on the frequency of false negative or false positive results in this field, but error is logically more likely to be recorded after false negatives, followed as they will be by the birth of a child with disability. Error is continually reported nevertheless, with false positives relatively high; over five per cent recorded in the most commonly diagnosed chromosomal abnormality, Down's Syndrome.

Screening tests are improving in accuracy but they still remain something of a lottery. The parents may be told that there is a one in 200 chance of something being wrong or it may be as high as one in ten. To the patient these odds may sound very frightening, but in effect mean that nine babies will be perfectly healthy for every one with disability. If termination is opted for after such calculations, many healthy babies will be killed.

The tests themselves may eventually become more accurate, but they will always rely heavily on the skill of the practitioner and of those who interpret the results. Some of the test procedures themselves carry risks. Amniocentesis has a one in 200 chance of causing miscarriage, which can make decisions very difficult for parents if they are also weighing up a one in 200 risk of abnormality. Earlier this year a report was published in Great Britain showing that four healthy babies miscarry for every Down's Syndrome baby detected. Professor Kypros Nicolaides, head of fetal medicine at King's College Hospital, London, commented in *The Sunday Telegraph* in April 2001:

> There has been an explosion in invasive testing since the 1970s. The incidence of Down's syndrome has not increased, but the number of tests has jumped from 3,500 to 40,000 a year, with an all-too-predictable loss of life.

It was revealed in 1995, that chorionic villus sampling (CVS), another invasive pre-natal diagnostic method, had actually caused serious developmental damage to at least 40 babies *in utero* in Great Britain and to 500 babies worldwide.

Neither does an initial diagnosis of abnormality tell you to what degree the individual child will be affected. Genetic counsellor, Barbara Biesecker, writing in the *British Medical Journal* (BMJ) in February 2001, points out that if a baby with Down's Syndrome has a severe cardiac abnormality, the prognosis will be completely different from that of a Down's child whose heart is unaffected. 'Healthcare providers can offer descriptions of populations of affected individuals, but no crystal ball exists for that particular fetus.'

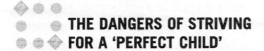

THE DANGERS OF STRIVING FOR A 'PERFECT CHILD'

Developments are not restricted to marking conventional diseases. Probably the most sensational offshoot of the Human Genome Project is the branch known as behavioural genetics, which claims that all manner of traits can be attributed to genes: aggression, criminality, homosexuality, intuition, hyperactivity are some which have hit the headlines. Already there are promises of eliminating undesirable traits, but experts warn that human behaviour will not be determined by single genes, but by complex interactions between environment and multiple genes. Techniques at the moment concentrate almost exclusively on the selective destruction of embryos and fetuses. How feasible is the transition from identifying and eliminating the 'defective' baby to designing the 'perfect' baby?

Some primitive attempts at enhancement are already in place. Designer sperm banks supplying superior products from Nobel Prize winners and other scholarly sources have been on the market for years and egg donors from Ivy League backgrounds are selling their gametes for upwards of $50,000. While the rules of the marketplace prevail in the USA, it is against the law in England for money to be involved in such transactions, but the search for superior genetic material goes on in this country nevertheless. An advertisement seeking egg donors appeared in the *Cambridge Alumni Magazine*, in Easter term 1999.

Embryo grading in IVF treatment, even without PGD, is another attempt to load the die towards the perfect child and assessment of the three-day embryo imposes a considerable degree of physical quality control. The process is explained in detail on the website of a fertility centre (www.advancedfertility.com) which notes that: 'Patients often ask whether low grade embryos will make low quality kids.' The answer assures us that: 'Children born from low grade embryos are just as cute, intelligent, strong, et cetera, as those born after transferring high grade embryos.' On that basis, then what is the purpose of the grading in the first place?

Couples have already chosen laboratory rather than natural conception in order to ensure the birth of a child with a specific type of genome. PGD was used in 2000 to find a sibling for a child suffering from Fanconi's disease, in order to obtain umbilical cord cells for treatment purposes. A Fanconi-free embryo, compatible with the sister's genome, was identified and other embryos were discarded. In 2001 in Rome, PGD sex selection was performed by doctors, not to avoid genetic disease but for a couple seeking to replace a dead female child. When only a male embryo was created, it was abandoned in the Italian clinic as the couple had four other sons and did not want any more. In both examples, the embryo was created as a means to an end, not respected as an end in itself.

REPRODUCTIVE CHOICE OR SELFISHNESS?

That is where we are today in reproductive technology. We can offer some degree of quality control but can guarantee nothing. Our approach is biased towards identifying (with serious margins of error) and destroying 'defective' embryos and fetuses rather than correcting or enhancing those we wish to improve. Our ability to design new life from scratch is very much in its infancy despite the revelations of the human genome. But the key question remains the ethical one: Should we be doing any of this in the first place?

Dominating the field of assisted reproduction is the ideology of choice, the so-called right to procreative liberty. This is presumed to flow automatically from the negative right acquired through the legalization of abortion. If there is a right not to gestate a child then it is argued that there is an equal right to gestate or gain access to a child through any means available. The rationale behind this position is rarely fleshed out and presupposes the acceptance of abortion in the first place.

American courts have avoided wherever possible any interference in procreative decisions, and in Great Britain the Human Fertilisation and Embryology Authority (HFEA), despite its empowerment by Parliament and numerous guidelines, in effect leaves most decisions to local ethics committees. The vague statement that by law nobody can be refused fertility treatment is frequently voiced by Mrs Ruth Deech, Chairman of the HFEA, although the public is very quick to express shock when another 60-year-old woman gives birth to twins by IVF or some tragedy follows a surrogacy agreement.

The easiest option in solving ethical dilemmas is to make a virtue out of unrestrained choice. But choices as serious as those involved in human reproduction must be made within a moral framework, so that we do not simply ask, 'What can I do?' but far more importantly, 'What should I do? What is right?' Science can add worthwhile technical dimensions to our lives but in this unique field new options are rarely morally neutral.

The ideology of choice comes up against a particularly serious obstacle when it endorses procreative liberty, insofar as the object of choice is no less than another human being. Both the abolition of slavery and women's emancipation were based on the truth that no person has a right to the possession of another person. Why should it be different for children? Public indignation at the excesses of assisted reproduction is usually centred on a perceived abuse of the rights of the vulnerable child: the right to autonomy, stability, information about genetic background and so on.

Three-times surrogate Claire Austin hit the headlines, 22 years after the arrival of the first test-tube baby, with a story involving almost all available reproductive technologies. A commissioning couple from Portugal and Italy, living in France, obtained eggs from an English donor and American sperm from a Danish sperm bank. Embryos were created in Athens to be carried by Claire, who returned to Spain. When it was discovered that the surrogate mother was carrying twin girls, the commissioning couple explained that they only wanted one boy, not two girls, and asked that the pregnancy be aborted. Claire was reluctant to do this and eventually the twin girls were given away to a lesbian couple living in Hollywood. Anthony O'Hear, Professor of Philosophy at Bradford University, voiced the concern of many when he commented that the story was one 'of astonishing human selfishness, muddle and unhappiness.... A story in which children are treated as if they were commodities or a sort of fashion statement' (*Daily Mail*, 8 May 2000).

The commodification of children in reproductive technology is turning parenthood into an unhealthy model of self-gratification rather than a relationship where unequivocal acceptance and love of the offspring, an ideal of previous generations of parents, is the primary focus.

◇ ● ●
● ● REPRODUCTIVE CHOICE OR
● ● ◇ EUGENICS BY STEALTH?

It is not just the child who is in a vulnerable position. Only the very naive can claim that those making reproductive choices exercise their rights in a totally objective context. Even adequate information and counselling can be a lottery. A study published in the *British Medical Journal* in February 2001 revealed enormous variations among different health professionals as to what they knew about sex chromosome anomalies and it was a matter of chance who passed the information on to patients after pre-natal testing. The authors concluded: 'It is disturbing to note the haphazard nature of how parents were informed of the diagnosis, what information was given, and what was implied.'

Surveys by groups such as the National Childbirth Trust indicate that many women feel pressurized into accepting scans and tests and finally abortion. Increasingly, women feel unable to refuse tests and screening in particular is presented as routine. Doctors and midwives claim that the search for the baby 'free of flaws' is parent driven, but parents complain that the opposite is true. 'Professionals will whisper helpfully that the birth of a Down's child is a life sentence which sensibly one should seek to avoid,' said Brian Wilson MP, father of a Down's Syndrome child, interviewed for *The Sunday Telegraph* in 1997.

Evidence of subtle coercion appeared over and over again in anecdotal evidence from a number of friends who have given birth recently. 'When I said I didn't want the transnuchal scan for Down's Syndrome,' said one mother, 'the ultrasonographer turned off the screen and wouldn't let me look at my baby. She was very cross.' 'I asked what a test was for,' said another colleague, recounting her experience of ante-natal care. 'Twenty anomalies,' she was told. When asked what these anomalies were and what could be done to cure them, the informant was unable to answer.

Utilitarian economics are freely expressed. The *British Medical Journal* regularly publishes articles where the costs of various ante-natal screening programmes are analysed and compared to the potential expenses involved in future healthcare were the pregnancy to continue. Having established that 'the cost of detecting a pregnancy affected by cystic fibrosis may range between pounds sterling 40,000 and pounds sterling 104,000,' one such article (December 1995) goes on to explain that their economic appraisal has adopted the most positive cost-benefit approach: 'For example, the avoidance of treatment costs incurred by an individual patient with cystic fibrosis (estimated in 1990 to be pounds sterling 8,000 a year for adults) may be seen as a large benefit.' 'Avoidance of treatment' should be translated into the less euphemistic 'termination of the pregnancy'.

While proponents enthuse about the application of the new genetics, others see ominous shadows of eugenics behind the current quest for the perfect child. Such accusations are usually denied by quoting the arguments for procreative liberty. It cannot be eugenics because it is not imposed by the state – pre-natal and preimplantation diagnosis are purely matters of parental choice. Apart from the issues of coercion just referred to, it makes no difference to the offspring whether it is killed by parental choice or state directive. It can even be argued that rejection by one's parents is actually worse for the child. The state is always accomplice in the act and the motivation is undeniably to eliminate the embryo or fetus with disability.

The word eugenics, from the Greek for 'a good birth', was coined by Francis Galton in 1883 and he defined it in a 1905 paper as 'the science of improvement of the human race germ plasma through better breeding.' Nowadays associated with Nazi extermination policies, eugenics developed initially in England and during the 1930s spread to America and Germany. Based on a desire for human perfection and a belief that 'the great majority of human beings are substandard' (Julian Huxley), the eugenicist's goal of selective breeding was achieved first by sterilization of those deemed inferior. By 1931 in America there were already 30 states with compulsory sterilization laws for 'so-called' sexual perverts, drug fiends, drunkards, epileptics and other diseased and degenerate persons.

The accent today may be more on eliminating physical rather than behavioural 'defects' and the technology may be more sophisticated, but the approach is hardly more subtle than it was in the past. Past-president of the American Association for the Advancement of Science, Bentley Glass, had no compunction in 1971 in stating that parents would in the future have no right 'to burden society with a malformed or a mentally incompetent child' and test-tube baby pioneer, Professor Robert Edwards, remarked at the 1999 Annual Meeting of the European Society of Human Reproduction that: 'Soon it will be a sin for parents to have a child that carries the heavy burden of genetic disease. We are entering a world where we have to consider the quality of our children.' But Cambridge History Professor, John Casey, in an essay in the *Daily Mail* (August 1997) warns us: 'People are naturally loath to draw connections between Nazi and communist ideas, eugenics, and what is now politically correct among the progressives. But there really is something in common: treating human life not as sacred and valuable in itself, but as a means to an end.'

Others are blinded to these obvious parallels. Professor John Burn, a leading UK geneticist, in a letter to *The Times* in June 1995, expressed his horror that compulsory abortion of abnormal children has become the rule in China and that sterilization of those with genetic disorders was being imposed on the carriers, describing this policy as the 'undisguised embodiment of eugenic principles'. His objections focus exclusively on the coercive element of the Chinese policy. However, the Chinese are simply further along a path that we are already marching along. The underlying principle, whether in sterilizing the adult or terminating the life of embryos or fetuses with genetic defects, is always to 'better' the human genetic stock.

Disability groups in the UK are in no doubt as to the discriminatory nature of genetic testing. 'The echoes of the Holocaust reverberate down the corridors of the genetics sector. Be warned, history can repeat itself. Geneticists plan for disabled people and other patients with gene faults to be dehumanised. We are to be ring-fenced as defective traits within the gene-pool' ('Fighting Back Against Eugenics...', Disability Action North East, 1998).

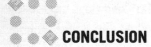

CONCLUSION

It is undeniably legitimate and perfectly normal for adults to wish for healthy offspring, but how this goal is realized is all-important and the child should always be welcomed for itself alone, not because it conforms to a model in the minds of its parents. Procreative liberty must not be dominated by the rights of parents in opposition to the welfare, let alone the very existence, of their children. The diagnostic tools of the new genetics are becoming more and more sophisticated in identifying genetic problems, but positive answers are minimal and there is little enthusiasm for developing cures; discarding the unwanted embryo and fetus is the preferred choice. This policy of destruction and discrimination add up to very bad medicine and immoral social policy and all our efforts and investment should be directed towards providing real cures which do not kill the patient. As new reproductive technology stands today, the old tradition which viewed the child as an 'accident of birth' to be accepted unequivocally, remains the best choice and is far more worthy of a just and civilized society than the current eugenic dream of designing perfect babies.

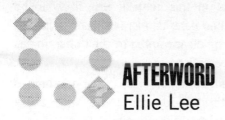

AFTERWORD
Ellie Lee

The essays in this collection suggest that answers to the question 'Designer babies: where should we draw the line?' rest on views about a prior question 'Are reproductive technologies, including PGD, dangerous or problematic?' In their essays, contributors to this book have set out a range of compelling and often competing arguments in response to this question. Some key points, which emerge from their discussions, can be summarized as follows.

YES, REPRODUCTIVE TECHNOLOGIES, INCLUDING PGD, ARE DANGEROUS OR PROBLEMATIC

Reproductive technologies such as PGD are substantially different from less sophisticated means through which parents attempt to influence their offspring, for example, taking folic acid during pregnancy. It is important to be cautious about these technologies, because the degree of control they offer in relation to choosing the genetic make-up of future generations introduces dangers in a range of areas:

1 Enabling parents to choose aspects of their child's genetic make-up is detrimental to the parent–child bond. It encourages the view that children are similar to commodities and should be judged according to whether they are of adequate 'quality' to meet their

parents' desires. Children are, in this context, less likely to be offered unconditional love by their parents, more likely to be judged and parents are more likely to be disappointed by their offspring as they fail to live up to their expectations.

1 Technologies that enable certain condition or traits to be 'screened out' encourage negative attitudes towards those with these conditions or traits and can lead to discrimination.

1 PGD and pre-natal screening as they currently exist are predicated in particular on negative attitudes towards disabled people. They rely on and encourage the idea that it is better not to be than be disabled and that pregnant women who opt to bear children with disabilities have made the 'wrong choice'.

1 The notion that individual choice should be the overriding criterion underpinning the regulation of reproductive technology needs to be challenged. The problematic implications of such technologies, as just detailed, make regulation necessary.

NO, REPRODUCTIVE TECHNOLOGIES, INCLUDING PGD, ARE NOT DANGEROUS OR PROBLEMATIC

The nightmarish scenario presented in much debate about 'designer babies' misrepresents the reality of what is possible. Many medical conditions and all character traits are complex and cannot be chosen or avoided through reproductive technology at present. Current debate is worse than inaccurate, however. It diverts attention from problems such as the high cost of treatment and lack of access to services for those who might benefit from, for example, PGD. Reproductive technologies offer significant benefits to those unable to conceive, who have a family history of genetic illness and who want to make a choice as to whether to bear a disabled child. Worries about these technologies are unfounded because:

1 The claim that children born as a result of reproductive technology are considered 'commodities' by their parents is unsubstantiated. This view is based on 'guess work', and it is problematic to traduce the kinds of relationships such parents have with their children in this way.

1 The argument that reproductive technologies lead to discrimination also has no basis in fact. Decisions made by individuals, when they opt to use such technologies, do not lead to diminished opportunities for others. No one else is harmed or has their opportunities in life diminished, where a potential parent opts to use PGD or other technologies.

1 While it is true to say that the provision of pre-natal screening and PGD may be predicated on concerns other than extending reproductive choice, this does not mean that they inevitably encourage negative attitudes towards disabled people. It is possible for ante-natal screening to be routine and for society to adopt positive policies towards already-born disabled people. Where individuals opt to use PGD, or choose abortion following ante-natal screening, it is wrong to imply they are anti-disability. While they may wish to have a child without a disability, this does not mean they have negative attitudes towards disabled people in general.

1 There are compelling reasons for defending an ethic of liberty in reproduction. Adults need to be able to make decisions about their personal lives and futures. Insofar as the decisions made with regard to reproduction do not harm others, people should be allowed to make them for themselves. This means that not only should people be able to use reproductive technology to avoid bearing a child with a disability if they so wish, they should also be able to use it to choose traits in their offspring, in the event of this being possible.

These contrasting approaches raise important issues regarding the regulation of reproductive technology. As outlined previously, at the current time access to treatments that involve human embryos, such as PGD, is regulated through clinical discretion. The clinician concerned judges whether it is 'in the best interests of the child' that treatment be provided to those requesting it. Decisions as to whether PGD should be made available in response to a specific request, for example to sex select, or to screen for a particular gene fault, is decided on a case-by-case basis.

Broadly speaking, at the time of writing, it has been considered ethically best so far to 'draw the line' at screening for non-medical reasons; that is, PGD is only offered to screen for a gene fault for a serious medical condition. Since February 2002, it is also deemed ethically justifiable in the UK to screen *for* certain genes – for example for those which can allow a future child to become a bone-marrow donor. In this instance too, however, the justification for this use of PGD rests on the criteria of medical benefit, although to an existing person, rather than to the child that may be born at a future point.

Some arguments made in this book present a challenge to this approach to regulation. Two key and competing approaches to regulation have been put forward. One argues, on the basis of an ethic of reproductive liberty, that regulation should be kept to a minimum. Access to PGD and other technologies can only be justifiably restricted where there is irrefutable evidence that use of the technology causes harm to others. In this scenario, if it were possible for potential parents to screen for traits, as well as medical conditions, they should be allowed to do so. The other contends that it is essential to regulate access to reproductive technologies strictly, on the grounds that they irrefutably damage parent–child relationships and lead to discrimination and anti-disability views. PGD might be allowed only for conditions that lead to early death. As the debate about where we should 'draw the line' continues, we hope these arguments will enable readers to judge for themselves whether and how law and policy need to change.

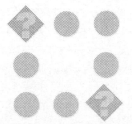

DEBATING MATTERS

Institute of Ideas
Expanding the Boundaries of Public Debate

If you have found this book interesting,
and agree that 'debating matters', you can
find out more about the Institute of Ideas
and our programme of live conferences and
debates by visiting our website
www.instituteofideas.com.
Alternatively you can email
info@instituteofideas.com
or call 020 7269 9220 to receive a full
programme of events and information about
joining the Institute of Ideas.

Other titles available in this series:

DEBATING MATTERS

Institute of Ideas
Expanding the Boundaries of Public Debate

TEENAGE SEX:

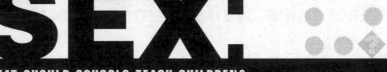

WHAT SHOULD SCHOOLS TEACH CHILDREN?

Under New Labour, sex education is a big priority. New policies in this area are guaranteed to generate a furious debate. 'Pro-family' groups contend that young people are not given a clear message about right and wrong. Others argue there is still too little sex education. And some worry that all too often sex education stigmatizes sex. So what should schools teach children about sex?

Contrasting approaches to this topical and contentious question are debated by:

- Simon Blake, Director of the Sex Education Forum
- Peter Hitchens, a columnist for the *Mail on Sunday*
- Janine Jolly, health promotion specialist
- David J. Landry, of the US based Alan Guttmacher Institute
- Peter Tatchell, human rights activist
- Stuart Waiton, journalist and researcher.

SCIENCE:

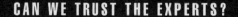

CAN WE TRUST THE EXPERTS?

Controversies surrounding a plethora of issues, from the MMR vaccine to mobile phones, from BSE to genetically-modified foods, have led many to ask how the public's faith in government advice can be restored. At the heart of the matter is the role of the expert and the question of whose opinion to trust.

In this book, prominent participants in the debate tell us their views:

- Bill Durodié, who researches risk and precaution at New College, Oxford University
- Dr Ian Gibson MP, Chairman of the Parliamentary Office of Science and Technology
- Dr Sue Mayer, Executive Director of Genewatch UK
- Dr Doug Parr, Chief Scientist for Greenpeace UK.

ART:

WHAT IS IT GOOD FOR?

Art seems to be more popular and fashionable today than ever before. At the same time, art is changing, and much contemporary work does not fit into the categories of the past. Is 'conceptual' work art at all? Should artists learn a traditional craft before their work is considered valuable? Can we learn to love art, or must we take it or leave it?

These questions and more are discussed by:

- David Lee, art critic and editor of *The Jackdaw*
- Ricardo P. Floodsky, editor of artrumour.com
- Andrew McIlroy, an international advisor on cultural policy
- Sacha Craddock, an art teacher and critic
- Pavel Buchler, Professor of Art and Design at Manchester Metropolitan University
- Aidan Campbell, art critic and author.

ALTERNATIVE MEDICINE:

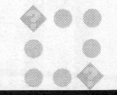

SHOULD WE SWALLOW IT?

Complementary and Alternative Medicine (CAM) is an increasingly acceptable part of the repertory of healthcare professionals and is becoming more and more popular with the public. It seems that CAM has come of age – but should we swallow it?

Contributors to this book make the case for and against CAM:

- Michael Fitzpatrick, General Practitioner and author of *The Tyranny of Health*
- Brid Hehir, nurse and regular contributor to the nursing press
- Sarah Cant, Senior Lecturer in Applied Social Sciences
- Anthony Campbell, Emeritus Consultant Physician at The Royal London Homeopathic Hospital
- Michael Fox, Chief Executive of the Foundation for Integrated Medicine.

COMPENSATION CRAZY:

DO WE BLAME AND CLAIM TOO MUCH?

Big compensation pay-outs make the headlines. New style 'claims centres' advertise for accident victims promising 'where there's blame, there's a claim'. Many commentators fear Britain is experiencing a US-style compensation craze. But what's wrong with holding employers and businesses to account? Or are we now too ready to reach for our lawyers and to find someone to blame when things go wrong?

These questions and more are discussed by:

- Ian Walker, personal injury litigator
- Tracey Brown, risk analyst
- John Peysner, Professor of civil litigation
- Daniel Lloyd, lawyer.

NATURE'S REVENGE?

HURRICANES, FLOODS AND CLIMATE CHANGE

Politicians and the media rarely miss the opportunity that hurricanes or extensive flooding provide to warn us of the potential dangers of global warming. This is nature's 'wake-up call' we are told and we must adjust our lifestyles.

This book brings together scientific experts and social commentators to debate whether we really are seeing 'nature's revenge':

- Dr Mike Hulme, Executive Director of the Tyndall Centre for Climate Change Research
- Julian Morris, Director of International Policy Network
- Professor Peter Sammonds, who researches natural hazards at University College London
- Charles Secrett, Executive Director of Friends of the Earth.

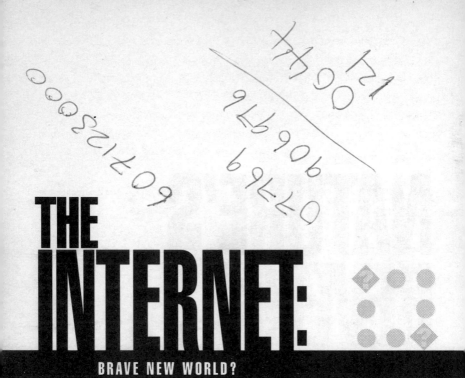

THE INTERNET:

BRAVE NEW WORLD?

Over the last decade, the internet has become part of everyday life. Along with the benefits however, come fears of unbridled hate speech and pornography. More profoundly, perhaps, there is a worry that virtual relationships will replace the real thing, creating a sterile, soulless society. How much is the internet changing the world?

Contrasting answers come from:

- Peter Watts, lecturer in Applied Social Sciences at Canterbury Christ Church University College
- Chris Evans, lecturer in Multimedia Computing and the founder of Internet Freedom
- Ruth Dixon, Deputy Chief Executive of the Internet Watch Foundation
- Helene Guldberg and Sandy Starr, Managing Editor and Press Officer respectively at the online publication *spiked.*